You Can Think Like a Psychiatrist

SECOND EDITION

You Can Think Like a Psychiatrist

SECOND EDITION

Leslie Lundt, M.D.

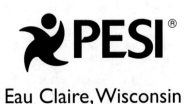

Eau Claire, Wisconsin
2009

ISBN: 978-0-98203-985-4
Previous ISBN: 0-9763885-0-2

Library of Congress Control Number 2005903453

Published by PESI, LLC
PO Box 1000
3839 White Avenue
Eau Claire, Wisconsin 54702

Printed in the United States of America

Think Like a Psychiatrist is intended solely for educational and
informational purposes and not as medical advice. Please consult a
medical or health professional if you have any questions about your
health.

Dr. Lundt has received research support from Cephalon, Eli Lilly,
Forest, GSK, Merck, Organon, Ortho-McNeil, Pfizer, Pharmacia,
Sepracor, Shire, and Targacept. She has participated as a consultant or
speaker for BMS, Cephalon, Eli Lilly, Forest, Genesis Pharma, GSK,
Janssen, Orphan Medical, Organon, Pfizer, Sanofi-Aventis, Searle,
Sepracor, Shire BioChem, Solvay, Takeda, and Wyeth.

Illustrations and cover design were created by Sean Fields.

PESI, LLC strives to obtain knowledgeable authors and faculty for its publications and
seminars. The clinical recommendations contained herein are the result of extensive
author research and review. Obviously, any recommendations for patient care must be
held up against individual circumstances at hand. To the best of our knowledge any
recommendations included by the author or faculty reflect currently accepted practice.
However, these recommendations cannot be considered universal and complete. The
authors and publisher repudiate any responsibility for unfavorable effects that result from
information, recommendations, undetected omissions or errors. Professionals using this
publication should research other original sources of authority as well.

For information on this and other PESI books, audio, and
video recordings, please call 800-844-8260 or
visit our website at www.pesi.com

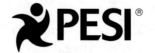

Dedication

This book is dedicated to our patients, who teach us more than we could learn from anyone else.

Contents

Tables

Illustrations

Preface

One of the most exciting things about studying medications that work in the brain is the rapid changes that occur. There are several new medications available since this book was first published in 2005. You will find information about these new options in this second edition.

Another major change is the focus of *Think Like a Psychiatrist*. The overwhelming cry that I heard when this book first was read by my colleagues was, "patients need to read this!" I wholeheartedly agree that in order to be a full member of the treatment team, the end-user (known as the patient) must be fully informed about how our medications work. You, too, can think like a psychiatrist.

Introduction

Canst thou not minister to a mind diseased,
pluck from the memory a rooted sorrow,
raze out the written troubles of the brain,
and with some sweet oblivious antidote
cleanse the fraught bosom of that perilous stuff
which weighs upon the heart?

—William Shakespeare

Half a millennium after Shakespeare wrote the above lines, professionals in mental healthcare continue to search for ways to help people plagued with mental distress.

In the following pages you will learn about medications that psychiatrists and others prescribe for people with depression, anxiety, sleeplessness and other conditions that arise from the way the mind works—or fails to work—as it should.

The information is presented from the perspective of a practicing psychiatrist, a medical doctor with special training and credentials in the diagnosis and treatment of children and adults with mental disorders.

I believe it's time for us psychiatrists to share our insights with the general public so that all of us can be blessed with enlightened perspectives in this rapidly changing arena of healthcare.

This book is your opportunity to learn to "think like a psychiatrist."

How a Psychiatrist Thinks

A middle-aged woman I'll call Sarah has finally decided to see her healthcare provider about her sleep problems, irritability, and moodiness. At the clinic she waits nervously for her turn in the consulting room.

Her thoughts ramble as she reviews the reasons she is there. Fatigue. "I'm always tired," she reminds herself. "And grumpy." Just that morning she remembers shouting, "Jeremy, get your shoes on—now! Now!" Her four-year-old scampered for cover under the dining room table where he struggled with his shoes. At the office later that day an assistant put papers on her desk for an important meeting, but a key document was missing. "I can't even count on you to carry papers from one office to another," she snapped.

It's been bad for her marriage, too. Sarah loves her husband Steve, but they've been arguing about everything. The discord reached such a tempo that they agreed they'd better see a marriage therapist to try to keep the relationship together. First, she's going to talk to her doctor.

"Sarah?" a voice calls out from the doorway from the clinic's waiting room. Sarah forces a smile and walks slowly to the office.

"You've got a bad case of depression," Dr. Toolley says after listening to Sarah describe her fatigue and her jumpiness. "I'm going to give you a prescription for some medicine that will help you with this problem. Take one of these every morning and come back in three months."

He hands her a prescription. It reads, "Paxil 20 mg."

Sarah dutifully takes the Paxil the next morning as directed. She feels even worse—sedated yet jittery and with a dry mouth. Reluctantly (not wanting to be a pest) she rings the office.

"You're experiencing some mild side effects," the nurse says. "That's to be expected with this medication, but they'll go away in a few days. You just hang in there, okay?"

The telephone clicks. "I shouldn't have bothered them," Sarah mumbles. "They're so busy."

She keeps taking the medication, but over the next several days Sarah becomes increasingly agitated and begins to have disturbing thoughts. One night she is sure she can't stand the noise from the barbecue going on next door. She fantasizes about shooting the neighbors. During the day she can't sit still at the office, and her feet are sore from blisters caused by endless pacing.

Afraid of what is happening to her, Sarah risks calling the doctor's office once again.

"I'll check with the doctor and call you back," the nurse says.

A couple of hours later the phone rings. It's the receptionist at the clinic. "The doctor has phoned in a prescription to your local pharmacy," the voice says.

At the drug store Sarah picks up the prescription, a supply of Ambien. The instructions and explanations the pharmacy attendant provides explain that the medicine is designed to help her overcome insomnia.

"Steve," Sarah complains that evening. "Now I'm on two different medications, and I don't like it."

"Hey, we're going to the marriage counselor tomorrow afternoon," Steve says. "Why don't you see what he says about this?"

"Good idea, honey."

The marriage counselor doesn't like what he's hearing. "I'm going to talk to my supervising psychiatrist," he says, "and see what she recommends. You're not getting the help you need."

The therapist discusses the issue with his supervising psychiatrist, who advises an immediate evaluation.

I have seen this scenario many times. A hasty diagnosis leads to the improper selection of medication. In Sarah's case, she was suffering from bipolar disorder, which was aggravated by the antidepressant Paxil. Soon she was on two different medicines—an antidepressant and a sleep aid—neither treating her primary illness.

Would Sarah have had more success in dealing with her depression if she had been equipped with a better understanding of how the brain works? Would she and her husband be able to deal with her symptoms if she could think more like a psychiatrist? What about her doctor? Would Dr. Toolley benefit from thinking like a psychiatrist, for example, considering all of the diagnostic possibilities after conducting the initial interview?

The best doctors focus on symptoms and consider every diagnostic possibility.

If he had, the doctor would have been focusing more on Sarah's symptoms than on her story. He would have considered each symptom before recommending a course of action.

Fortunately for Sarah and Steve, their marriage therapist played a pivotal role in reversing near disaster by questioning Sarah's treatment course. Once she was on the right medication for her problem, her symptoms of fatigue and agitation subsided, and she was able to move ahead with her life.

Sarah was lucky. Some patients wait even longer for an appropriate diagnosis and treatment, and many who could have responded positively to a course of treatment never receive the relief they need to put their lives back together.

This book will help people like Sarah and her husband sense when the care provider is not dealing with the real issues and to know the appropriate steps to take.

If you or a loved one has suffered from a severe emotional disturbance, you may have witnessed first hand the turbulence of moving from institution to institution won-

The challenge is helping people deal with difficulties beyond comprehension.

dering what the next day will bring. After years of being handed around from one form of treatment to another before achieving success in overcoming deep-seated problems, a patient of mine put it this way: "I now have a life that is manageable. Stability is so important to me. For the first time in my life I feel like I can count on what will come in the future."

To achieve success like that is a reward worth working for. The specialized training and experience psychiatrists possess give them insights that cut through myths and mis-understandings related to mental health. As a family member or close friend of someone afflicted with mental health problems, you can provide priceless support.

You can become a patient partner, someone who knows enough about medication to question the doctor about prescription choices or to watch for interactions and side effects. You can share details that the doctor may never ask for, and in this way help the doctor identify the disease process and recommend the best course of action for alleviating the symptoms.

If you are the victim of these problems yourself, you face the challenge of learning to think like a psychiatrist so that you can apply advanced insights into living and working with mental disorders.

An army of caregivers

Let's continue our journey into the world of psychiatric treatment by visiting the bustling—if imaginary—Take Care Primary Care Clinic.

The clinic is located in a typical corner of America, and Take Care doctors see patients with a variety of ailments and health problems. Most of their patients have a mental health component to their illness, and for some of them the decision to see their doctor was driven by their anxiety, depression, or some other mental state that disturbs them. In other words, like Sarah, they come to Take Care clinic for mental healthcare.

One mental healthcare provider in 1,000 is a trained psychiatrist.

Take Care clinic is situated in a metropolitan area with a population of about half a million people, so we can assume that there are ten to fifteen board-certified psychiatrists available to diagnose mental illness, prescribe medications, admit patients, and manage mental healthcare for patients who seek their services. There are probably another fifty to one hundred psychologists and therapists offering a variety of mental health services, and scores of clinics such as Take Care representing hundreds of healthcare professionals who are involved in the treatment of mentally ill persons.

We haven't mentioned the nurses and other staff members at mental health hospitals or psychiatric wings of hospitals or the swelling ranks of "alternative care" therapists who offer everything from incense to massage for healing the mind and calming the soul.

Nor have we mentioned parents and teachers, who have a huge influence in the care and upbringing of children, including those with serious mental disorders.

This is a huge army of caregivers.

For every professionally trained psychiatrist there are probably a thousand or more who are providing mental healthcare of one kind or other to children, teenagers, adults, and the elderly. As a practicing psychiatrist associated with a thriving mental health clinic, I am fully aware of the tremendous level of assistance my patients receive from healthcare experts and others in the community where I live and work.

This book is dedicated to the proposition that many of the observational and treatment skills that we psychiatrists master during our training and experience should be freely shared with the millions of people who receive or are involved with people who receive psychiatric services. The consumers who take the medications prescribed for them need a better understanding of how those medications work and their potential for harm as well as relief.

You won't become a psychiatrist by reading this book, but my hope is that you will find in these pages many of the the key principles and facts that make good psychiatry work so well.

You can help build bridges to primary care doctors and psychiatrists. Your alertness to sound psychiatric principles will help you know how to access the level and type of mental healthcare needed most.

You can learn to think like a psychiatrist.

Principles of Prescribing Psychiatric Medicines

What is it like to achieve success in the battle against mental disorders? One patient described it this way: "It was a transformation, from feeling shame—Is this a punishment for something I've done?—to getting recognition for my accomplishments. Too many mentally ill people are seen as society's feared minority. I am no longer intimidated by this classification. No matter what I've gone through, I'm still the same loving, kind person I was before. I'm no longer afraid of being diagnosed. When you come down to it, I'm not substantially different from others."

This brilliant young man was fortunate because he was able to obtain the level of care he needed to give him a productive role in society. Appropriate medication was a major factor in his success.

We begin the study of psychotropic medications, the term for medicines used in psychiatric treatment, with a brief look at the basic premises a psychiatrist uses in choosing the most effective medications for the treatment of mental disorders.

There are no magic bullets

The first principle we need to absorb when we look at psychotropic medicines as a psychiatrist does is that there are no magic bullets. Let me state this more emphatically:

Not one psychotropic pill is capable at any dose for any length of time of curing even one person.

Unlike many physical problems, disorders of the mind are not caused by an intruder such as a virus or infection that can be disabled, destroyed, or sidelined. The psychiatrist cannot run a lab test to identify the type of mental problem and then prescribe a course of treatment that will eliminate the disease. There are no easy targets and no magic bullets in psychiatric medicine. This is a major barrier in treating mental illness.

We treat symptoms, not diseases

The second reality we all need to face is that because we cannot precisely define or diagnose mental illness, all we can do is address the symptoms. Accepting this fact can be humbling, but accept it we must. Even if the medications we prescribe decrease pain and improve mental function, they do not cure. They only alleviate the symptoms, and they only work as long as they are in the blood stream. Stop taking the medicines, and their effects also stop. Being unable to prescribe a cure can be extremely frustrating to care providers if their training and experience have taught them to identify the cause of disease and prescribe medicines and therapy to promote the restoration of health. It's a harsh reality, but in the world of mental health there are no sure cures.

> **As soon as a person stops taking the medicines, any benefits also stop.**

Medicines affect the whole body

A complicating factor in treating people with mental disorders is the fact that the medicines prescribed for such conditions do not stay in the brain. They circulate throughout the body, affecting every body organ they touch and modifying every body function.

Even neuropharmacologists do not fully understand why certain medications cause side effects such as sexual problems, weight gain, tremors, or insomnia, but they know they do. The mechanisms in the brain that bring about the benefits of psychotropic medicines are just as baffling.

We should be concerned about the power and complications associated with the medications prescribed to help people deal with psychiatric problems.

One patient, a variety of possibilities

Dozens of valid ways of evaluating and treating a patient are available today. When I present a lecture to psychiatrists, I often show a video of one of my patients (with their permission, of course). I am always amazed that in a room of twenty doctors, there may be fifteen different treatment approaches suggested to deal with that patient's mental disorder.

For many patients there is no simple path to follow. The best course often involves a combination of treatment modes such as exercise, balanced nutrition, "talk" therapy, and medication.

Names are overly simplistic

"We think in generalities, but we live in details."

Alfred North Whitehead probably wasn't thinking about psychotropic medications when he made the above comment, but designer brand names and marketing messages don't reflect the essential details about these important agents. We are guided too often by all-encompassing promises rather than the details we need for a valid evaluation.

For starters, the generalized labels assigned to classes of medications do not fully describe how they are used. Antidepressants, for example, are used not only to treat depression, but also to blunt the symptoms of anxiety, eating disorders, pathological shopping, gambling, and even some kinds of sexual dysfunction. Antipsychotic medications are prescribed to treat anxiety, insomnia, and impulsivity as well as hallucinations and delusions. Off-label uses further multiply the application of drugs developed and approved by the FDA for specific purposes.

> **Labels do not fully describe the ways medicines are used.**

Conditions cross boundaries

The process of identifying and naming a category of mental illnesses such as anxiety, depression, or bipolar personality unbundles a host of interrelated symptoms and contributing factors. A person with bipolar disorder, for example, may be depressed much of the time and feel anxiety, although mania is the most celebrated of the person's symptoms. Categories may be necessary, but they do not completely describe all of the symptoms of any of the persons whose problem is labeled.

Often patients have more than one mental disorder, and selecting the best medication becomes even more important. "One of the first doctors I saw about my problems diagnosed OCD (obsessive compulsive disorder)," a patient told me, "but totally missed the bipolar. So I got the wrong medication, and this slowed down progress considerably."

Start low, go slow

Early in their training psychiatrists learn to "start low and go slow" when prescribing psychotropic medications. In other words, the doctor learns that it is best to prescribe the very lowest dose expected to have a positive effect and then gradually increase the dosage throughout the course of treatment. This approach is a guiding principle in the treatment of patients by psychiatrists.

We want to prescribe the lowest dose that may have a positive effect.

Why not do it the other way around? Why not speed things up by prescribing the maximum amount of medication so that we can observe the most phenomenal results?

The answer is "side effects." These are the unwanted consequences of absorbing drugs into the bloodstream. All drugs create side effects. We not only want to avoid those that are irritating, such as dry mouth or a mild headache, but also those that may be harmful to the body, such as increased blood pressure, heart irregularities, and rashes.

Side effects are often surprises. Nobody expected that the erection-enhancing drug Viagra would cause some people to see the world with a bluish tint because the drug distorted their color perceptions. Depending on the person's job and other lifestyle issues, this effect could range from a minor annoyance to a serious consequence of taking the drug.

An antipsychotic drug called Zyprexa often causes weight gain, possibly by slowing metabolism and heightening a person's desire for fattening foods. A patient diagnosed with schizophrenia may do well on Zyprexa from a psychological perspective but gain a hundred pounds in the process.

Like Zyprexa, many other psychiatric medications also result in weight gain.

"Wait a minute," you may be saying. "I can hear the problem already. I know a person who is depressed because she's fat. You're saying by filling a prescription for antidepressant medication, she will gain weight. How in the world is that going to help her?"

Your concern is justified. The "cure" may be more harmful than the disease. A person who is depressed because she's overweight needs a combination of treatment methods to help her address her weight issues in addition to treating her for depression.

The patient defines the problem

Think about the last time you paid a visit to your healthcare provider. More than likely, you were weighed, and somebody took your temperature, measured your blood pressure, and noted your heart rate. The doctor asked you some questions and after a brief exam may have ordered blood tests and perhaps even an X-ray, CAT scan, MRI or other diagnostic tests.

No objective test can identify a mental disorder.

For mental disorders there is no reliable battery of laboratory tests that can make a diagnosis. Lab tests that are ordered sometimes help the provider know what is going on in the patient's body, but for the most part, providers rely on the patient's own interpretation of what is going on.

The psychiatrist may help patients describe their discomfort by completing forms consisting of long lists of symptoms to check off. A check mark, of course, is only an indication of what the patient sensed when completing the form. There is no second opinion, no back-up test, no way of verifying the accuracy of the check marks. The resulting checklist is only a subjective evaluation by the patient. The person filling out the form decides what his or her symptoms are—not the doctor.

This may seem an indirect way to inquire about mental functioning, and it is. Checklists, however, can be a relatively simple way to evaluate how mental problems are affecting the individual.

Weigh the benefits

Like all prescription drugs, psychotropic medicines are powerful chemicals that affect the whole body. In this book we will talk about many unwanted side effects that occur when drugs that offer the promise of a healthier life are taken. The careful psychiatrist always considers key factors related to the course of treatment before writing the prescription and handing it to the person.

- Is the known risk of side effects worth the expected benefits from the medicine?

- Has the person ever been treated with this medication? If so, what was the response?

- Is there a family history of using this medication? How successful has it been?

- Can the cost of treatment be covered by the patient, the family, or insurance?

- Does the selected medicine have a good chance of being taken as prescribed or will the patient reject it for any of the above reasons?

When you think like a psychiatrist, you will weigh the benefits against the risk of side effects for any psychotropic medication that may be prescribed or recommended. The psychiatrist's decision about what to prescribe and appropriate dose levels for the medication must be based on a careful analysis of the benefits and the possible side effects for each individual.

Be prepared to wait

The amount of time it takes for psychotropic medication to take effect varies widely from drug to drug. Imagine someone you know who suffers from panic attacks and sees a psychiatrist. If an antianxiety drug is prescribed, fifteen minutes after taking it, the patient will feel better. An antidepressant drug, on the other hand, may take four to six weeks before it begins to work. Medications for obsessive compulsive disorder may not take full effect for months.

Medicines may take weeks to take effect.

When you "think like a psychiatrist," you will realize that there are many different timelines for the medication prescribed to help patients. Sometimes it takes patience while you wait (and wait) for results.

Taper on and taper off

Another mindset to cultivate in order to "think like a psychiatrist" is to be aware of what happens when a person's medication is discontinued. Unwanted symptoms, known as discontinuation effects, may occur. The rule, "Taper on and taper off," applies to any medication affecting the brain. The doctor who follows this guideline doesn't want to prescribe a promising drug only to be surprised by dangerous side effects that make the medicine intolerable.

People want to be well

You won't find it in any pharmacy, but probably the most effective medicine of all is the inborn desire by persons afflicted with mental illness to reach a state of equilibrium so that they can resume a normal life.

As a person concerned about the workings of the brain, your mission is not merely to look for ways to patch up the breaks and bruises but also to help individuals grow strong in self-reliance and good mental health.

I continue to be amazed at the resilience of the human spirit.

Working with Primary Care Practitioners

As powerful and complex as psychotropic medications are, most are prescribed not by mental health specialists but by primary care providers.

The fact that the primary care provider has scores of resources at his or her fingertips doesn't always guarantee that the best course of treatment will be chosen. Problems or limitations can arise when a family depends on a primary care practitioner to guide the care of persons with psychiatric disorders.

Underdosing

Doctors in family practice and other branches of medicine may not be fully trained in the pharmacology of these complex medications. They often know just enough to be aware of the possibility of serious side effects or other unfavorable consequences, and out of a reluctance to risk bringing these on, they tend to underdose.

The problem is that while a small dose may help the person avoid side effects from many of these drugs, too little too late is even worse. This type of caution doesn't help the patient feel better.

Another possible problem when primary care physicians prescribe medications for mental health problems is the scant amount of time spent evaluating the individual's needs. The average amount of

Average time with a primary care physician— 5 minutes or less.

time a primary care physician spends one-on-one with a patient is less than five minutes per office visit. Too often the office visit consists of a brief conversation followed by a prescription or a sample packet handed to the patient with a quick, "Try these." The evaluation of the treatment's effectiveness is left up to the patient.

The patient has probably learned about the medications the doctor prescribes from television, acquaintances, and other sources. It's understandable why the patient feels like a failure because the medications seem to help other people but not him or her.

Long lapses between visits

Another fact you need to remember about the relationship between the typical primary care provider and a mental health patient is that the primary care doctor tends to see each patient only rarely. The interval from the start of treatment to the next follow-up visit may stretch on for months.

This is a natural consequence of what is going on in the doctor's life. They are pressed for time. The scheduling routine needed to maximize their billing potential too often leaves patients with the impression that their concerns don't matter. As a result, patients sometimes gloss over serious problems that need to be addressed. For other patients, the stress associated with a doctor's visit may cause them to forget what they intended to tell the doctor. Still others feel ashamed to tell the whole story, especially since they're sure the doctor is pressed for time.

If only patients could realize how effectively their pain and suffering could be treated, they would not hesitate to let the doctor know what is troubling them.

If someone you care about needs help with these issues, you may be able to fill a role of encouraging that person to achieve a fuller level of mental health and vigor. You will probably spend far more time with the person than the prescriber will, and this can give you a better sense of the scope of the problem. You can help bridge the gap caused when people sense that the doctor is very busy. You can take the time to go with the person to the doctor's office or coach the person ahead of time so that they won't hold back information out of fear of complaining too much. You can urge the patient to be honest in describing discomfort when the doctor asks how they're doing.

You can encourage the relative or friend who knows and trusts you to tell the doctor what is going on and suggest ways to communicate their needs more effectively, such as making a list of problems or keeping a diary with short descriptions of symptoms. You can help divert them from the tendency to go to the doctor with a smile pasted on their face, minimizing symptoms and saying, "I'm fine," "Everything's okay," and "Couldn't be better."

Another tip is to suggest that the patient place his or her concerns in writing. Remind the person that brevity is the key to getting a doctor's attention. Doctors will read brief and relevant letters or notes, and the letter will be in the patient's chart when the next visit occurs. From both a medical and a legal perspective, there's no better way to remind the doctor of important issues. Your written note is hard to ignore.

However limited the time with the doctor may be, the patient has direct access to the doctor, and the doctor will listen to the patient. This can place the burden for describing and even treating the illness on the patient.

Perhaps you would guess that I think all people with mental health problems should be under the care of a board-certified psychiatrist. Not so. As with all medical specialties, psychiatry is not always the perfect setting for dealing with personal problems. It takes time to open up, to share perspectives, to develop trust so that the psychiatrist's words of advice will be taken seriously.

Over time you can usually build a relationship of mutual trust with the primary care providers so that your observations will be taken seriously.

When that happens, everybody wins.

Working with Psychiatrists

You are fully qualified as a caring person to work with a psychiatrist in clarifying a treatment plan or discussing how you can assist a patient on the road to recovery. Don't let the classification of being an "ordinary person" keep you from being involved with the psychiatrist in caring for the patient.

Or, if you are a patient, consider yourself a partner with the psychiatrist in seeking solutions.

What are psychiatrists anyway? What should you know about them so you can help someone struggling to benefit from psychiatric help?

Help patients communicate better with their doctor.

Psychiatrists are first of all physicians, medical doctors who have chosen to specialize in the diagnosis and treatment of individuals with mental disorders. They have studied the human body and have a solid understanding of how it functions from a purely physical perspective. They have also taken special training in most medical specialties such as obstetrics and gynecology, cardiology, dermatology, and surgery.

Psychiatrists have a huge respect for the human brain and for the way it handles millions of messages simultaneously. They have spent an enormous amount of time in the classroom and continue to attend seminars learning all they can absorb about the neurological system.

Psychiatrists are also avid students of the fascinating world of psychotropics, the primary subject of this book. Every practicing psychiatrist has seen families and individuals rescued from unspeakable horrors and people restored to productive, satisfying lives because of the miracle of modern pharmaceuticals.

Psychotherapy—"talk therapy"—is also used effectively by psychiatrists, who are often in a unique position to combine both forms of treatment: psychotherapy and medications.

Unfortunately, psychiatrists do not exist in sufficient numbers to evaluate or treat even a significant fraction of the people whose mental health depends on the quality of care they receive.

You may not be a psychiatrist or a professional healthcare provider, but you can help a loved one with mental health problems take the steps they need to take to lessen their symptoms and enjoy a better state of mental health. If you are seeking help for your own mental health problems, you will want to freely share information with your therapist or counselor so that he or she can do a more effective job of advising you. You may also want to enlist the support of a family member and friend who has read this book or has special training in listening to troubled individuals. This person can direct you to a therapist qualified to meet your special needs.

A psychiatrist is a physician with special training in how the human mind works.

The best therapeutic situation, of course, is one in which the patient is motivated to get better and will have enough insight to help the primary care physician or psychiatrist make appropriate treatment decisions. The patient who is determined to alleviate the symptoms of a mental disorder has a good chance of doing just that.

When you engage the services of a psychiatrist, don't be surprised to learn that ten-minute visits are not unusual.

This may be twice as long as the primary care physician typically provides, but it isn't enough time for a thorough evaluation of what is going on. You may want to search for a therapist who can spend more time with you so that your treatment will be more complete.

No two psychiatrists are alike, of course, and you won't necessarily find one who is able to relate to you in a helpful way. Unfortunately, even psychiatrists can easily slip into a mood of apathy. Perhaps you've heard of the patient in therapy who bursts out, "People don't give a hoot about anything I say," to which the psychiatrist quietly responds, "So?"

> **Every day the psychiatrist faces competing interests.**

For their part, psychiatrists are bombarded by dozens of competing interests. One of the most pervasive is the notorious formulary, a list of medications that qualify for insurance coverage. This is a particular barrier with managed care systems. If a drug the doctor wants to prescribe is not on the list, it may not be covered even though it may be a better choice for the patient.

The psychiatrist also faces pressure from varying standards and diagnostic trends in the local psychiatric community. In one city, for example, the diagnosis of bipolar disorder is the most popular; in another it could be depression or anxiety. Like it or not, psychiatrists are influenced by their peers in the practice of their specialty.

A good psychiatrist will welcome the thoughtful participation of the patient and trusted friend in the evaluation and treatment.

The Search for the Perfect Pill

"They (drug companies) have too much control over the evaluation of their own products, and that's a conflict of interest."—Marcia Angell

*J*ulie is depressed. Matthew is failing math. Grandpa Henderson can't remember what happened five minutes ago. Mom is worried sick about almost everything in her life. The neighbor's kid went on a rampage and is no longer allowed to attend high school.

No cause for alarm. For each of these unfortunate conditions, there's a pill–a magic pill to calm the angry, re-orient the confused, inspire the listless, and bring hope to the discouraged.

You know all too well that it isn't that easy. If it were, crime as we know it would have ceased to exist long ago. Nobody would be sad. We would all get perfect grades in school, and everybody would get along with everybody else.

Psychotropic medications are a $20 billion industry.

If we don't live in a perfect world, it's not because the drug companies aren't trying. A whole new class of medications has been developed to deal with troublesome moods and other mental problems. The use of psychotropic medications is climbing rapidly.

Antidepressants, one category of psychotropic medications, are now a twenty billion dollar industry in the U.S. A 1997 study showed that nearly eight out of ten persons being treated for depression received some kind of psychotropic medication as part of their treatment.

The money is well spent from the perspective of thousands of people who live relatively normal lives as a result of these and other medications that affect the way the mind functions. Many owe their lives to modern advances in psychopharmacology. As a psychiatrist, I marvel at the way these brain-influencing drugs can restore hope to the troubled. I have seen youngsters whose extreme hyperactivity was threatening to destroy a classroom reverse their behavior and go on to be helpful members of the class after taking a prescribed course of medication.

I have also seen the relentless course of Alzheimer disease halted in its tracks when someone began taking medication that may not cure, but at least can slow the progression of this debilitating mental disorder.

And nothing is more rewarding than seeing a teenager trade a cloak of despondency to one of "can-do" optimism due at least in part to a careful course of antidepressant medication.

Imagine how wealthy you would be if you could sell a product that millions of people would use every day for years. This is the hope for every new drug that is developed and the reason that doctors are continually being urged to prescribe specific medications. To help persuade them, pharmaceutical firms that develop and manufacture drugs spend a major share of their advertising dollars on the medical community.

Drug companies try to persuade physicians to prescribe their medicines.

As a result, doctors receive a huge amount of information from drug companies about the benefits of various prescription drugs. Besides sharing data, these companies also attempt to win friends among doctors by giving away mementos such as logo-inscribed pens, calendars, note pads, coffee cups, caps, golf tees, and many other low-cost items.

It adds up fast. The January 1999 edition of the *Journal of the American Medical Association* reported that pharmaceutical companies spend an average of $8,000 to $11,000 per year on each practicing physician to promote their wares.

Drug companies don't stop with tangible objects bearing the name of the drug being promoted. A quieter but much larger phenomenon is the presentation of meetings and medical journals funded solely by pharmaceutical firms.

The information presented at these classes and seminars is usually not junk or advertising hype, but solid, scientific data. Drawbacks and side effects involved in every drug are clearly presented. Details about research required to convince the Federal Drug Administration to approve the drug are freely shared.

Without the pharmaceutical companies covering the cost, the medical community might not be able to afford to hire the top medical experts in the world to present the seminars that physicians attend free.

I am not embarrassed to admit that I've been to beaches and mountain resorts, Europe, and many other places to attend meetings of leading doctors from around the world–expenses paid by leading pharmaceutical houses. I am treated well. More importantly, I learn a lot and am able to interact with psychiatrists from around the world.

To avoid compromising their principles, some doctors will not attend these seminars. Some even refuse pens or other items imprinted with a message touting the benefits of a certain medication. I would love to live in a world where I could obtain all the data I need from sources with no financial interest in the success of their products, but I can't. The reality is that you can't escape the influence of pharmaceutical companies that are providing this data.

Drug companies fund nearly all the studies needed for acceptance by the FDA. They then recover the cost of research and development of new drugs by selling billions of pills and other medications.

Drug companies present valid data at seminars.

Sales representatives who call on doctors to show them the latest wares offered by a pharmaceutical company provide one of the most persuasive ways to influence prescription habits by physicians.

Sometimes the influence of even one pharmaceutical rep who is sold on the effectiveness of a specific drug and possesses great selling skills can boost the number of prescriptions for that medication. I remember learning about a certain antidepressant drug that suddenly became extremely popular in one area of the country. A researcher who came across the data decided to find out why. It turned out that in one county, a female pharmaceutical rep was faithfully making the rounds at physician offices selling the drug with the outstanding record. She was bright, persuasive–and drop-dead gorgeous.

In her book, *The Truth About Drug Companies,* Marcia Angell, a former editor of the *New England Journal of Medicine,* estimates that pharmaceutical companies spend two and a half times as much on marketing and administration as they do on research. Dr. Angell has little sympathy with the way drug companies manage the production, approval, and marketing of their products.

The quote I've selected for this chapter from Dr. Angell about drug companies having too much control over the evaluation of their own products, which is a conflict of interest, comes from an interview by MotherJones.com with the Foundation for National Progress in September 2004. The hard reality is that, like every other corporation in the country, drug companies are in business to make money. Their profits make it possible for them to develop innovative new treatments.

I do not see a built-in conflict between serving the health needs of the public and operating a financially viable business. Nobody wants to turn the calendar back to the days when the mentally ill were warehoused like animals or when depression was a hidden plague.

What we need today is not fewer drugs but a greater understanding by all of us in the use of psychotropic medicines. The more we know about how our body absorbs and utilizes these drugs, the better we can understand the effect these powerful medical substances can have on how we think and feel.

Let's widen the circle of understanding.

There is no lack of data. Pharmaceutical companies develop mountains of knowledge as they conduct research involved in the production of new medications. Doctors who are continually studying new advances in pharmacology are also a gold mine of information about how their patients respond to various treatment modalities.

It is time to widen the circle of understanding beyond the professional circles of those whose careers depend on patient care. It's time to deliver a solid set of information about the treatment of mental disorders to the patients themselves as well as their family members and close friends.

For whatever reason you chose to open this book, I suggest that you place the highest priority not on absorbing the facts presented in these pages but by learning to "think like a psychiatrist." The facts follow that purpose.

So much for a quick overview of some of the issues involved in prescribing drugs for people with emotional and psychiatric problems. In the next chapter we will look at the brain itself, where signals originate that determine how we feel and behave.

How Does our Brain Work?

Although the adult brain weighs only about three pounds, the spongy sphere of "gray matter" encased by a shield of bone is complex system that processes information, sends and receives signals, makes us happy or sad, and keeps us alive.

Chemical reactions gone awry in the human brain plague millions of children and adults today. Psychotropic medications zero in on these chemical reactions to provide relief.

The control center in our brains manages about one hundred billion brain cells–neurons–that are the building blocks of our brains. Neurons dart through the brain sending messages or signals to specific locations in the brain.

Our neural network has 10,000 X 100,000,000,000 connections.

Neurons do not touch each other directly but rely on a chemical reaction triggered by bursts of electrical energy to transmit messages. Each neuron uses an average of ten thousand connections to send one signal to another neuron. Multiply ten thousand connections times one hundred billion neurons, and you begin to get a picture of the enormity of the network within our brains.

The messengers that deliver messages within the brain are chemicals known as neurotransmitters. We have over sixty neurotransmitters in our brain. Neurons are continually assessing the need for more chemical products and, through a complex network of commands and activities, hundreds of powerful drugs emerge in our brain to help keep us functioning at optimal levels.

Neurotransmitters are chemical agents that are manufactured by the body from amino acids. They have two primary functions: to excite or to inhibit. Their role depends on the type of receptor cells at the destination where the message is delivered.

Newly made neurotransmitters immediately go into a mode of readiness, waiting in super-microscopic bubbles called vesicles for their first work assignment. The connection between neurons is known as a synapse. Think of the synapse as a tiny moat or transition point between two neurons. Synaptic vesicles are packed with neurotransmitters waiting to be deployed.

For a particular message to make a successful trip between neurons, one of the two neurons is configured as the sending neuron and the other as the receiving neuron. When the sending neuron receives a message to prepare for action, the vesicle pops open, like a balloon pricked by a pin. The neurotransmitter is released and floats into the space of the synapse. Of course, it can't do any good just floating around, and even if the neurotransmitter might prefer a life of leisure, hungry enzymes in the synapse are waiting to devour it.

The brain doesn't want to let disasters like that occur. In less time than you or I can imagine, the receptor site on the receiving neuron sucks the neurotransmitter in, rather like a pinball being pulled into its hole.

But not always. Through a process called reuptake, the neurotransmitter is sometimes sucked back into the first cell where it remains in storage. Think of this as a self-stocking refrigerator that brings food back into itself.

The drawing below gives a simplified picture of how the process of sending messages from one neuron to another works.

In this drawing you can see the axon, a protruding section of a neuron, and a bulge at the end of the axon where the neurotransmitters wait for their next signal ordering them to travel to another neuron. To reach their destination, each neurotransmitter has to travel across a very small gap, or synapse, to the dendrite, the receiving part of the neuron that serves as a miniature reception center.

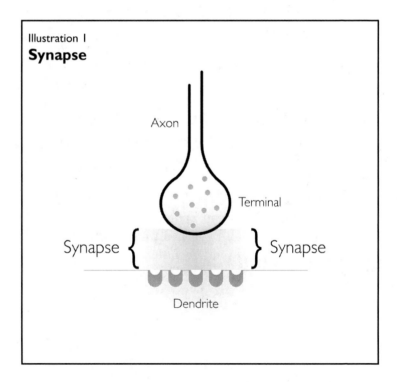

Illustration 1
Synapse

Axon

Terminal

Synapse { } Synapse

Dendrite

The illustration below gives another perspective of how the neurotransmitters become activated. You can see a group of neurotransmitters waiting in containers called "synaptic vesicles" for their traveling orders.

Across the gap (synapse) you can see receptor cells in the dendrite portion of the neuron that has been selected as the destination. Each neurotransmitter must reach the appropriate receptor in order for the message to be conveyed accurately.

Once the receptor cells in the target neuron have received the chemical message from the neurotransmitter, they are deactivated so that they can receive the next message. All of this takes place with blinding speed. Like keys

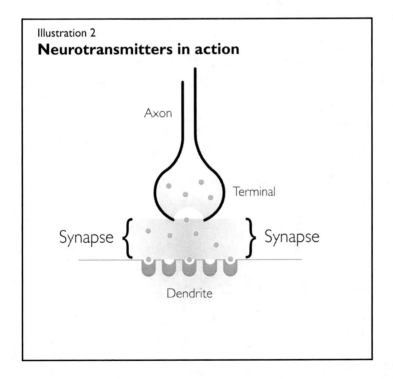

Illustration 2
Neurotransmitters in action

Axon

Terminal

Synapse { } Synapse

Dendrite

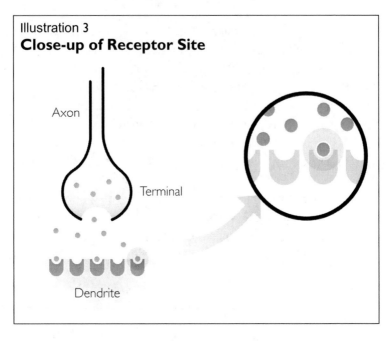

Illustration 3
Close-up of Receptor Site

Axon

Terminal

Dendrite

in a lock, the messenger neurotransmitters are recognized by the receptors in the membrane. See Illustration 3, above.

Types of neurotransmitters

Three types of neurotransmitters have been identified:

- Classical neurotransmitters

- Neuropeptides

- Soluble gases

Classical neurotransmitters

The term "classical" when applied to neurotransmitters refers not to their design but to the fact that they were

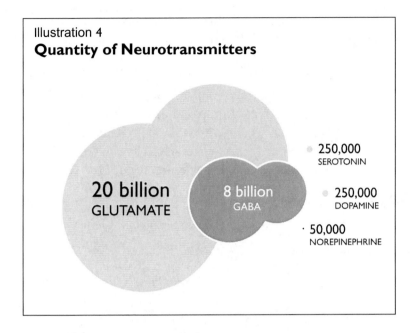

Illustration 4
Quantity of Neurotransmitters

20 billion
GLUTAMATE

8 billion
GABA

250,000
SEROTONIN

250,000
DOPAMINE

50,000
NOREPINEPHRINE

discovered first. Most classical neurotransmitters were identified in the first half of the twentieth century.

For an idea of how many of these neurotransmitters are
busy at work in our brains, consider the following numbers:

- Glutamate system: More than 20 billion
  cortical neurons, mostly excitatory

- GABA system: 8 billion cortical
  neurons, mostly inhibitory

- 250,000 dopamine neurons

- 250,000 serotonin neurons

- 50,000 norepinephrine neurons

As you can see, by far the most common neurotransmitter in the brain is glutamate, a chemical in the category of "classical" neurotransmitters.

You may recognize this chemical from the term "MSG" for monosodium glutamate. Glutamate is valued by chefs and manufacturers of prepared meal items for its ability to enhance flavor. The use of MSG in prepared foods is a subject of some controversy, since one to two percent of the population has a severe allergic reaction to MSG.

Glutamate "steps on the gas."

More than twenty billion of our body's neurons use glutamate, a "step on the gas" substance that helps get things moving. In chemical terms, glutamate is an "excitatory neurotransmitter." Glutamate is also valuable as a regulator of memory and cognitive learning.

The second most common neurotransmitter is also in the "classical" category. For simplicity's sake, GABA is known by its initials rather than its full name, gamma amino butyric acid. GABA sends messages to eight billion neurons in the brain, acting in an opposing way to glutamate. While glutamate stimulates and excites, GABA calms and slows down. It is the most inhibitory transmitter known.

GABA regulates feelings of anxiety and our ability to sleep. Medicines that increase the supply of GABA are prescribed to treat anxiety and sleep disorders. Alcohol and tranquilizers also tend to stimulate the activation of GABA in our brain.

In our discussion of GABA we've been talking in billions. Now we're going to move down the scale to numbers that are microscopic by comparison.

Dopamine and serotonin each have 250,000 neurons in its domain. Norepinephrine, another neurotransmitter, has only 50,000. As insignificant as these chemicals may seem when compared to the vast quantity of neurons associated with glutamate and GABA, these chemicals are more familiar to people and are influenced by many of the psychotropic medicines we prescribe.

Peptides

The second category of neurotransmitters are peptides, the "new kids on the block." More evidence is needed to define these chemical messengers of the brain more accurately.

Neuropeptides, or just "peptides" in this discussion, are much larger than the classical or "small molecule" neurotransmitters. They consist of three to sixteen amino acids, while classical neurotransmitters have just one amino acid molecule.

"Molecules of emotion" is the way one neuroscientist, Candace Pert, chose to describe peptides in her book by that title.

Peptides— "Molecules of Motion"

Of all the peptides, we probably know more about the one called Substance P than any of the others. Substance P transmits messages triggered by pain. If you are feeling pain, it's because Substance P has signaled your brain.

You might conclude from the above explanation that the "P" in "Substance P" stands for "pain," but it doesn't. An amusing explanation for the "P" is that it is an abbreviation for "pee," where the substance was first discovered. Who said that biochemists don't have a sense of humor?

As important as the pain signal from Substance P may be, Neuropeptide Y is the most common peptide in the brain, and it seems to play a major role in obesity. In controlled studies, laboratory rats injected with this neuropeptide quickly gained weight. Scientists are still studying the implication of these and other studies to learn possible ways of dealing with Neuropeptide Y to control the threat of obesity for a huge fraction of the population.

Beta endorphins are peptides that come from the pituitary and seem capable of producing a greater sense of exhilaration than all the other excitatory endorphins.

Neurokinins are a class of peptide neurotransmitters associated with the promotion of stress and anxiety responses, the transmission of peripheral pain signals (similar to Substance P), and the modulation of opiate reward systems. Recent preclinical and animal models have suggested that neurokinin antagonists may have a number of clinical applications in the disruption of these systems.

These are just a few of the fifty peptide neurotransmitters that have been identified.

Soluble gas neurotransmitters

Some scientists place all neurotransmitters in two categories: classical or neuropeptides. However, today we're paying more attention to a third category of hard-working messengers, soluble gas neurotransmitters.

The best known of these is nitric oxide, which has the effect of increasing blood flow by dilating blood vessels. This is the mechanism that causes a man's erection. Viagra enhances the effect of nitric oxide by blocking certain enzyme systems that contribute to its destruction.

How neurotransmitters affect emotions

Most people assume that serotonin is the most prevalent neurotransmitter because they hear so much about its role in antidepressants. They are wrong. Serotonin is a small and scarce chemical in the "classical" category. It regulates anxiety, mood, and appetite. Drugs that act on serotonin are used as antidepressants and as medications to treat persons with anxiety and eating disorders.

Serotonin kicks in after a Thanksgiving feast.

Think of how you feel after Thanksgiving dinner. The serotonin you added to your body's brain chemistry makes you calm, full, a little sleepy, not wanting sex. Too much serotonin can lead to a sense of sedation and a loss of sexual desire—a continuation of the satiated feeling that comes after a Thanksgiving feast.

Dopamine is a neurotransmitter with a similar effect of boosting moods. It increases a person's ability to concentrate and helps him or her feel motivated to stick to a task. Even more important in our drug-abusing culture is the role of dopamine as the "reward chemical." A surge of dopamine in the brain causes a feeling of accomplishment. The energy and sense of reward from the release of dopamine triggered by cocaine encourage the user to dope up again and again. The reward is so intense that you can become addicted to cocaine after just one use. Other drugs of abuse, including amphetamines, also give the user a "high" by stimulating the release of dopamine.

Usually a transportation molecule returns the dopamine to the neuron where it came from, but a dopamine-enhancing drug such as cocaine prevents this round trip from occurring, so dopamine builds up, and intense feelings of pleasure result.

The body has a self-regulating mechanism to deal with too much dopamine. As the concentration of dopamine increases, the neurons with dopamine receptors produce fewer and fewer of them until dopamine levels return to

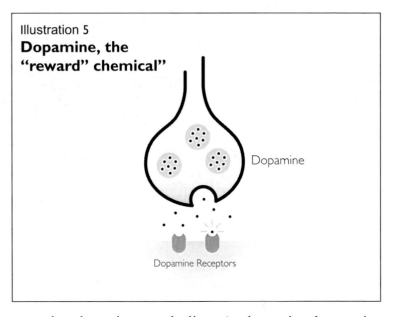

Illustration 5
Dopamine, the "reward" chemical"

Dopamine

Dopamine Receptors

normal and continue to decline. At that point the cocaine user feels a desperate need to restore dopamine levels by taking more cocaine.

Dopamine drugs are used clinically to lessen symptoms of ADD (attention deficit disorder) and certain disorders that cause persistent fatigue. Another medical application of dopamine is in treating Parkinson's patients, who have trouble with movement because they are short on dopamine.

The chemical compound acetylcholine is a neurotransmitter also used in treating Parkinson's Disease. Acetylcholine takes the honors as the first neurotransmitter to be identified and described by biochemists. It is not a drug in itself but regulates our attentiveness and memory. It also plays a role in helping us achieve deep, restful sleep.

The neurotransmitter norepinephrine stimulates the part of the brain that controls moods, energy, alertness, and the ability to pay attention. The famous "fight or flight" response to surprise is triggered by norepinephrine. The chemical also enhances alertness, concentration, and energy. Too much norepinephrine and you feel anxious or panicky even when there is no reason.

Epinephrine is another name for adrenaline, and you will sometimes see norepinephrine called noradrenaline, especially in the UK.

Antidepressants

All of us feel blue at times, but major depression results in profoundly dark moods frequently marked by uncontrolled crying, low energy levels, difficulty concentrating, and poor motivation to get things done. Suicide is an ever-present risk.

The primary medical goal for these people is to see symptoms disappear or at least take on manageable proportions. The good news is that antidepressants can do their job effectively. Despite this, controlled trials to evaluate the effectiveness of antidepressant medications indicate that only thirty percent of depressed persons experience full remission of symptoms when they complete a course of antidepressant medication.

Many persons treated for depression suffer from insomnia, fatigue, and other symptoms of depression that persist even after successful treatment with antidepressants. Another disappointment is that the class of drugs known as antidepressants do not immediately take effect. A person can't go to the drugstore feeling depressed and discouraged, get the prescription filled, take a pill or two and be contented and happy by the end of the day. A fast track for a demonstrable difference after a person starts taking antidepressants may be several weeks.

Several weeks is a fast track for antidepressants to take effect.

Not only that, but things may get worse before they get better. Before any benefits of the medication are noticeable, side effects have probably already taken over.

This means that the mental healthcare provider needs to see the patient being treated for depression several times early in the course of treatment. Frequent visits help the therapist monitor side effects and encourage the person to comply fully with the program outlined. For children and adolescents being treated with antidepressants for the first time, the FDA now suggests weekly visits with the prescriber.

FDA suggests weekly visits for children taking antidepressants.

If the medication does not have the needed effect, the dose may be increased beyond standard levels. This is because needs vary widely from person to person. Some do well on extremely low doses while others need to exceed even the maximum dosage set by the FDA to experience the desired effect.

Too often a primary doctor who lacks extensive training in psychiatric medicine will simply hand the patient a sample packet provided by the drug company. This approach can be futile because without close observation of the patient at regular intervals, the doctor cannot determine the effectiveness of the prescription or the appropriate dose. As a result, a doctor may keep refilling the prescription without increasing the dose as long as the patient requests refills. When complaints emerge about symptoms of depression or side effects such as sleep problems or fatigue, the doctor may discontinue the prescription prematurely.

Choosing an antidepressant

As psychiatrists, we begin the selection of an appropriate medication to treat depression by identifying the neurotransmitters we think are involved. Then we seek medicines that act on those neurotransmitters, either to stimulate or suppress them, and prescribe accordingly.

Every antidepressant drug currently being prescribed works on at least one of the following neurotransmitter systems:

- Serotonin

- Dopamine

- Norepinephrine

In choosing an antidepressant we often try to link specific symptoms to either an excess or a deficiency of dopamine or norepinephrine. Then we choose a prescription drug based on our impression of what the target neurotransmitters may be. Although this is a highly oversimplified method, it serves as a jumping-off point to help us choose among over twenty different antidepressants.

The next step is to consider side effects that could develop or worsen due to the circulation of antidepressant medications in the bloodstream. Finally, we look at the patient as a whole person and evaluate the depression in the context of other health problems, severity of symptoms, past history dealing with depression, and other factors.

We do not want to make things worse for the depressed person. If a fashion model comes for help with depression, for example, we won't be helping her by prescribing medication that will make her gain weight. We could wreck her career, and she'll have more problems than she did when she made an appointment to see a psychiatrist. Or what about the depressed patient who reports being sluggish and sleepy most of the time? A calming antidepressant is the last thing that person needs.

Cost is inevitably a factor in making the choice of an antidepressant. A person with medical insurance may find that the policy does not cover the cost of these prescriptions.

Since some medications will cost up to $100 or more per day, the patient's ability to pay needs to be considered when we recommend a course of treatment.

As a last resort, if the depression is severe and the patient is not responding to the medication, electroshock therapy (ECT) may be considered. When I was a student in medical school, ECT was much more common than it is now. Today there is no option for ECT in some cities, where local laws prohibit the procedure. Even where it is permitted, ECT carries a huge stigma. Still, it remains an excellent option for the profoundly depressed individual.

Other factors that affect depression

The above barriers to treatment may be alarming, but there are other factors that can interfere with a person's progress in dealing with a mental disorder

Medicines. As surprising as it may seem, some medicines can actually *cause* depression. A leading example is a family of drugs known as "Benzos," for benzodiazepine. Others include Beta blockers like Inderal (propanolol) and Catapres (clonidine), two drugs that are used to treat blood pressure, and steroids—especially progesterone and cortisone, and the Parkinson drugs l-dopa and Sinemet (carbidopa-levodopa).

Physical illness. You should also be aware that some illnesses can cause depression. Low blood pressure, anemia, AIDS, mononucleosis, pancreatitis, Cushing disease, infectious hepatitis, multiple sclerosis, and influenza are examples of physical conditions that can magnify or lead to severe or prolonged depressive symptoms.

Hormones. Some women become depressed because of the state of flux of their hormones. This happens on a monthly basis for many women. Pregnancy, birthing, and menopause are other times when female hormones can trigger depression.

Lack of sunshine. You may know someone who is profoundly affected by depression according to the time of year. Seasonal Affective Disorder, or SAD, is the name given to a gloomy or depressed state that can take over during the winter when there is less sunshine in the northern climates. Families living close to the Arctic Circle often invest in elaborate artificial lighting systems to keep from submerging into a joyless state when darkness prevails as much as twenty or twenty-two hours a day. I often suggest less extreme measures to my patients such as using a phototherapy box or a dawn simulator, combined with a wake-promoting medication.

Drug interactions. The prescribing doctor needs to know the names and dosages of all prescription and non-prescription medications the depressed person is taking because antidepressant medicines can interact with them.

One of the most popular drugs of all is alcohol, which can react dangerously with prescription medications, including those taken for depression and other emotional problems. One of my patients asked me to share with you the following plea:

"Understand that psychotropic medications do not mix with recreational drugs or alcohol. You can end up with a deadly poison if you ignore the interactions of these chemicals." —A patient

Side effects of antidepressants

Side effects, or unintended consequences, of taking an antidepressant usually occur during the six weeks or more it takes for the medication to work optimally in the system. During this time the patient needs to be monitored frequently in order to encourage full compliance and to monitor side effects. It is hard for most people to imagine a course of treatment that starts out with a burst of good feelings and then plunges into a course of uncomfortable side effects that can make them feel worse than before. Nevertheless, it is one possible outcome when a person is being treated for depression with prescribed medications.

The side effects can make a person feel worse than before taking the medication.

Another major problem often encountered by patients being treated with antidepressants is a negative effect on sexuality. When you think like a psychiatrist, you are aware of unwanted effects or lack of response after the individual begins taking the medication.

If the person is responding but only partially, anticipate a change in medication or an increase in the dose. A prescription may be supplemented with another medication, such as a sleeping pill for the person whose antidepressant medication is causing sleep problems. These changes should be made only when there is enough evidence to justify an alteration in the course of treatment.

Taking antidepressants with food is the best way to reduce the risk of negative effects. Taking a sedating medication at bedtime can also help the person obtain needed sleep if the drug causes restlessness.

Antidepressants and neurotransmitters

Since depression may be triggered by chemical signalling deep in the brain, it shouldn't be a surprise to learn that anti-depressant medications focus on neurotransmitters, the communication chemicals of the brain. Specifically, most antidepressants affect serotonin, norepinephrine, and dopamine.

Maybe you've seen the cartoon by Gary Larson with the unfortunate person at the gates of hell confronted with two choices: "Damned if you do," reads the sign on one door. The other door is labeled, "Damned if you don't."

Antidepressants are like that. There is no guarantee that all the consequences of following a prescribed course of these medications will be good ones. Negative effects vary according to which neurotransmitter—serotonin, nore-pinephrine, or dopamine—is affected.

We also need to remember that when we start talking about antidepressants, we are not only dealing with specific neurotransmitters but also with the way they interact with each other.

Serotonin. Side effects from antidepressants that work on serotonin include sexual dysfunction, stomach upset, and sleep disturbances. These occur because drugs that stimu-late serotonin are associated with a lack of libido and inabil-ity to have orgasms. Increased serotonin is linked to sexual problems in more than half of all people taking this class of drugs. Sleep disturbances are also common, as is stomach upset.

When the medication suppresses messaging by seroto-nin, the person may not be able to sense pleasure and may feel listless and unmotivated to do anything. A shorter attention span and problems remembering or using information may also result.

Serotonin antidepressants may also suppress the action of dopamine, resulting in difficulty in concentrating.

A subtle but potentially disabling side effect of antidepressants acting on serotonin can be the total relief of sadness without any other benefits. The person taking this type of antidepressant is not depressed but may express a lack of feeling and say "It's okay. Nothing matters." These people truly do not care what happens—and that is not a desirable outcome. We call it apathy.

Norepinephrine.
Medications that work on the norepinephrine neurotransmitter can lead to dry mouth, tremors, rapid heartbeat, difficulty sleeping, feelings of being anxious, and higher blood pressure.

Dopamine.
Uncontrolled movement of the hands and feet or "tics" and unwanted blinking or jerking of small muscles are disturbing side effects of this kind of antidepressant. Existing psychoses may also be aggravated by antidepressants using the dopamine mechanism.

Another side effect of drugs that stimulate the dopamine neurotransmitter may include a wound-up, restless, nervous state. The person can't sit still. Abnormal muscle movements, or tics, are not common but may occur.

The following table summarizes how serotonin, norepinephrine, and dopamine affect our moods.

How Neurotransmitters Affect Moods

	Serotonin	Norepinephrine	Dopamine
Anxiety	X		
Appetite	X		
Alertness		X	X
Motivation			X
Energy		X	X
Muscle movement			X
Concentration		X	X

A psychiatrist will start with the symptoms, determine which neurotransmitters are most closely associated with those symptoms, and then choose a medication that will work on the selected neurotransmitters.

MAO inhibitors

From time to time you probably see a warning stating that patients taking MAO inhibitors should not take a certain medication. What are MAO inhibitors and why do they cause problems?

MAO = an enzyme that attacks the mood-altering neurotransmitters.

The acronym MAO in the term "MAO inhibitors" represents mono-amine oxidase, an enzyme that is capable of attacking mood-altering neurotransmitters in the brain such as serotonin, dopamine, and norepinephrine and rendering them dysfunctional. Drugs that interfere with these attacks are known as MAO inhibitors.

In the 1950s an orthopedic surgeon named David Bosworth began prescribing iproniazid, an MAO inhibitor. His patients were not suffering from depression, but were veterans at a U.S. tuberculosis sanitarium. The drug had been found to be effective in the treatment of tuberculosis.

A delightful "side effect" of the drug was the happy feeling that the recovering patients experienced. Scientists had discovered that MAO inhibitors are able to control the activities of nerve receptor proteins that make us happy or sad. People taking mood-boosting MAO inhibitors were feeling good. A miracle drug was born.

Before long pharmaceutical houses were manufacturing and packaging MAO inhibitors, and people were taking them as antidepressants.

The three original brands of MAO inhibitors are Nardil (phenelzine), Parnate (tranylcypromine), and Marplan (isocarboxazid).

In Canada and Europe a different type of MAO inhibitors are known as Reversible Inhibitors of Monoamine, or RIMAs. The most popular drug in Canada in this class is Manerix (moclobemide), known as Aurorix in Europe. RIMAs are distinguished from the older MAOIs by their selectivity and reversibility. As a result, dietary restrictions are not required.

MAOIs are no longer considered the miracle drug for treating depression.

MAO inhibitors are especially useful in treating a form of depression marked by such characteristics as increased sleep and appetite, anxiety, and sensitivity to rejection. This problem is known as atypical depression because at first the medical community thought it occurred only rarely. Now we know that atypical depression is quite common, especially in women.

THINK LIKE A PSYCHIATRIST

As the years went by we discovered that there *are* side effects of taking MAO inhibitors, including weight gain, insomnia, and sexual dysfunction. By far the most serious problem is the risk of a life-threatening interaction between these drugs and foods containing the amino acid tyramine.

MAO inhibitors allow tyramine levels to build up in the body. Tyramine affects blood pressure, and in the most deadly situation, the chemical reaction of tyramine and an MAO inhibitor can increase blood pressure until it blows out a person's blood vessels and causes a major stroke. This is more than an abstract fact to me; I have had two patients who had serious medical consequences because of the death-dealing mixture of tyramine and an MAO inhibitor.

Antidepressants (MAOIs)

Relative Adverse-Effect Profiles

Agent	Usual Adult Dosage (mg/d)	Drowsi- ness	Sexual Dysfunc- tion	Agitation/ Insomnia
Nardil (phenelzine)	45-90	moderate	very high	low
Parnate (tranyl- cypromine)	30-60	low	very high	high

Adapted from CNS News Special Edition December 2004

Although tyramine is present in many foods, we only need to be concerned about its possible reaction with an MAO inhibitor when a large amount is present. Foods that have aged or contain a lot of yeast are candidates. Be sure to counsel a patient taking MAO inhibitors as antidepressants to avoid high-tyramine foods such as sour beer, aged cheese, aged wine, fava beans, smoked meats, sausage, beef and chicken livers, and packaged soups.

Unfortunate side effects can also result when MAO inhibitors are taken by people who are taking antihistamines and certain cold medicines.

Demerol is a popular pain medication that can produce deadly results when taken with MAO inhibitors. I remember clearly, as if it happened last week, the death in a hospital's emergency department of a person who died because of the interaction between Demerol and an MAO inhibitor.

Patients with prescriptions for an MAO inhibitor are more common in New York City because some psychiatrists in that city have vast experience with these drugs, allowing them to have less fear of their potential dangers. Outside of New York City, you will rarely encounter someone on these medicines.

Demerol and MAOs can be a deadly combination.

Emsam is the newest antidepressant released in the U.S. and the first patch for the treatment of Major Depressive Disorder. Selegiline, the active ingredient in Emsam, has been used for the treatment of Parkinson's disease. Clinical trials have shown significant improvement in depressive symptoms using this monoamine oxidase inhibitor (MAOI). A whole new generation of psychiatrists is being introduced to this very effective medication with a new delivery system.

Through transdermal (through the skin) delivery, Emsam is directly and continuously absorbed into the bloodstream over a 24-hour period. As a result, initial exposure of the drug to the digestive tract is minimized. The Emsam patch allows for levels of medicine to inhibit MAO-B in the brain thought to be necessary for antidepressant effect while sufficiently preserving MAO-A in the digestive tract to break down tyramine.

This means that at lower doses we do not have to worry about the dietary restrictions as we do with older MAOIs. To reduce the risk of blood pressure problems, dietary modifications are required with higher doses (Emsam 9 and 12 milligram patches). Foods and beverages high in tyramine must be avoided while on Emsam at these doses and for two weeks following discontinuation of Emsam, just as in older MAO inhibitors.

The most commonly reported side effect in clinical trials was skin irritation.

Tricyclic Antidepressants

The normal cycle for a neurotransmitter's work as a chemical messenger begins with receiving the message. Then it moves the message across the synapse to the receptor site on a welcoming brain cell. Immediately the neurotransmitter is sucked back across the synapse to the waiting rooms (vesicles) on the other side.

The class of antidepressants known as tricyclic drugs get in the way of this recycling activity. Specifically, they block the return (reuptake) of the neurotransmitters serotonin and norepinephrine back to the presynaptic neuron.

A single daily dose of a tricyclic antidepressant (abbreviated TCA) can often relieve a depressed person from dark moods and reduce the risk of panic attacks. It may take as long as eight weeks before the drug begins to take effect, and side effects almost always occur before the positive benefits are felt. Uncomfortable side effects that may occur include dry mouth, constipation, urinary retention, dizziness, sexual dysfunction, sedation, and weight gain. Irregular heart rhythms occur rarely, and deaths resulting from cardiac irregularities associated with use of tricyclics have been reported.

Although the two main uses of tricyclics are to relieve symptoms of depression and alleviate pain, the drugs are sometimes prescribed to treat attention deficit hyperactivity disorder (ADHD), cataplexy (sudden loss of muscle tone), nightmares, post-traumatic stress disorders (PTSD), sleep terrors, sleep walking, separation anxiety, migraine headaches, and insomnia. The FDA has approved tricyclic antidepressants for the treatment of depression as well as bed wetting among children.

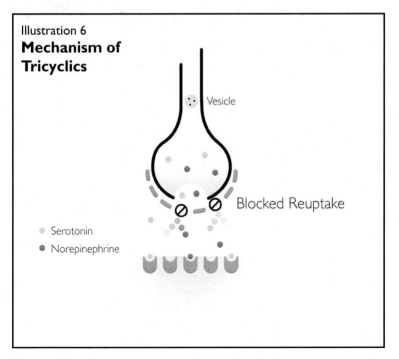

Illustration 6
Mechanism of Tricyclics

Vesicle

Blocked Reuptake

Serotonin
Norepinephrine

Elavil (amitriptyline), Aventyl and Pamelor (nortriptyline) are the tricyclic antidepressants most commonly prescribed for pain.

Other examples of tricyclics prescribed today include the following—

Norpramin (desipramine)

Sinequan (doxepin)

Tofranil (imipramine)

Surmontil (trimipramine)

Although for several years the benefits of TCAs made these drugs popular with patients and their providers, the sky darkened when consequences of overdosing became apparent. Resulting heart problems, including irregular rhythms, can be fatal. Even as little as one week's worth of meds can lead to death. Writing a prescription for a tricyclic antidepressant is like handing the depressed person a loaded pistol.

Tricyclic Antidepressants (TCAs)

Relative Adverse Effect Profiles

Agent	Usual Adult Dosage (mg/d)	Drowsiness	Sexual Dys-function	Agita-tion/ Insomnia
Anafranil (clomipramine)	100-250	high	high	none
Aventyl Pamelor (nortriptyline)	75-150	moderate	high	very low
Elavil (amitriptyline)	50-200	very high	high	none
Norpramin (desipramine)	100-200	low	high	very low
Sinequan (doxepin)	75-200	very high	high	none
Surmontil (trimipramine)	50-150	high	high	none
Tofranil (imipramine)	100-300	high	high	low
Vivactil (protriptyline)	15-60	low	high	high

Adapted from CNS News Special Edition December 2004

The increased risk of heart failure and suicide has turned many mental healthcare providers away from using tricyclic antidepressants.

Years ago doctors used these medications because they were simpler than shock therapy, and they were all that were available.

Tricyclic antidepressants are still used frequently by primary care doctors and pain clinics to help patients cope with chronic pain and occasional insomnia, but they have largely fallen out of favor with psychiatrists.

SSRIs

Waiting in the wings was the development of a new breed of antidepressants known as SSRIs (selective serotonin reuptake inhibitors). These drugs work on the mechanism that recycles the serotonin neurotransmitter after it delivers its message to the receptors across the synapse. SSRIs block the return (reuptake) of serotonin back to the presynaptic cells.

An early theory explaining depression was that serotonin seems to be lacking in depressed persons. The work of SSRIs in slowing down the recycling process was seen to cause more serotonin to be present at the receptors in the post-synaptic neuron, thus reducing symptoms of depression.

An interesting benefit of SSRIs is that they are not affected by alcohol as much as are tricyclic antidepressants. They are also much easier to tolerate, take effect with only one dose per day, and do not cause many of the side effects that made tricyclics so uncomfortable.

The first SSRI on the market was Prozac (see page 60) followed by Zoloft (sertraline), Paxil (paroxetine), Luvox (fluvoxamine), Celexa (citalopram), and Lexapro (escitalopram). Anafranil (clomipramine) combines the features of a TCA and an SSRI.

The FDA has approved prescriptions for SSRIs to treat a wide variety of mental disorders. Some of the most common ones are the following—

- Major depressive disorder

- Premenstrual dysphoric disorder

- Social anxiety disorder

- Post traumatic stress disorder

- Panic disorder

- Generalized anxiety disorder

- Bulimia nervosa

Once the FDA approves of drugs for specific problems, they are often prescribed for other conditions as well. This is called "off-label" use because it is not included in the official product information provided by the FDA. An estimated 80 percent of psychiatrists' prescriptions are "off label" in one way or other.

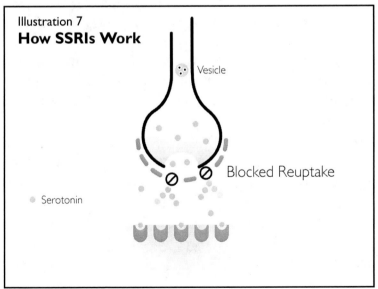

Illustration 7
How SSRIs Work

Vesicle

Blocked Reuptake

Serotonin

Off-label uses of SSRIs include treatment of premature ejaculation, compulsive behaviors such as gambling and obsessive shopping, separation anxiety, and simple phobias.

As helpful as SSRIs may be, patients taking them may experience side effects such as nausea, short-term anxiety, tremor, lack of libido or ability to achieve orgasm, weight gain, difficulty falling asleep or waking up, cognitive problems, and apathy. This may seem like a formidable list, but most patients are able to tolerate these problems. Also, many of the side effects diminish with time.

A warning from one parent on the use of SSRIs:

"Watch out for psychologists and psychiatrists who play roulette with meds. If one SSRI didn't work, they'd pull out another one. When the prescribed drug didn't give immediate results, they doubled the dose." —Concerned parent

Approximately two to three percent of persons taking SSRIs experience an immediate, intense, and negative reaction. The possible association between SSRIs and suicidal behavior continues as a topic of debate by scientists.

The benefits apparently outweigh the drawbacks, because drug companies continued scrambling to introduce the world to new SSRIs.

Prozac

Everybody loved the miracle drug Prozac (fluoxetine) from the moment it arrived on the horizon in January, 1988. Advertising assured the public that one size would fit everybody. Just one 20 milligram dose a day of this drug, and depression was history. At least, that's how the story went.

With aggressive marketing by manufacturer Eli Lilly, Prozac reached the pinnacle of psychotropic medicine within two years as the most prescribed antidepressant medication in the world. Prozac became a household word.

It is indeed good news that the risk of death from an overdose of Prozac is almost nonexistent. The rate of death for persons taking Prozac is less than one per million prescriptions, while tricyclic antidepressants and related drugs are associated with nearly 35 deaths per million prescriptions.

Prozac quickly became the most prescribed antidepressant.

The popularity of Prozac was phenomenal. "I want to kiss the person who invented Prozac!" was the theme of many who finally found relief from their nagging depression. Prozac seemed to provide the ideal solution to those longing to follow the "Don't worry, be happy" mantra that had never seemed to materialize for them before.

Heavy advertising catered to the swelling demand of people seeking not so much a cure for depression as a quick route to "feeling good." A positive benefit of the meteoric rise in popularity of Prozac was a relaxing of the stigma formerly attached to all forms of mental distress. Being depressed became socially acceptable now that Prozac was waiting to ease the discomfort.

Several best-sellers dealt with the promise of Prozac, including *Listening to Prozac,* by Dr. Peter D. Kramer, who wrote the following summary of how the drug was received:

"Prozac seemed to give social confidence to the habitually timid, to make the sensitive brash, to lend the introvert the social skills of a salesman."

Eli Lilly was basking in its success with Prozac and preparing to launch a new version of the wildly popular drug when dark clouds appeared on Prozac's horizon. Investigative reporting led to disturbing revelations.

As early as February 1992 Martin Teicher and Jonathan Cole, both highly respected American psychiatrists, published a paper in the *American Journal of Psychiatry* noting that six patients treated with Prozac developed "intense, violent, suicidal preoccupations" after starting the medicine.

A report printed by the *Boston Globe* on May 7 of 2000 stated that the drug company had changed the wording of physician reports about how well Prozac had worked for their patients. Instead of "suicide attempts," the documents were altered to read "overdoses," and instead of "suicidal thoughts," the word "depression" was substituted. Lilly was also accused of failing to reveal the refusal by the German equivalent of the FDA to allow the drug into that country. The decision was made because of findings concerning its use by patients who were not suicidal. For these patients the rate of suicide and suicide attempts was *five times* higher than for those taking older antidepressants and three times higher than for those taking placebos.

A major newspaper reported that documents were altered.

Lawsuits emerged naming Eli Lilly as the defendant in murder or suicide cases. Prozac was blamed for the suicide of pop music star Del Shannon and for the brutal murder of a woman in Maui and the suicide of her husband, who had been taking Prozac for two weeks. Multiple cases such as these began attracting media attention.

The Prozac issue became a huge hot potato in medical politics. The medical profession felt so comfortable with the drug that physicians whose practice included depressed individuals went into a state of denial. The consensus among these professionals and others was that the rare suicide attempts following Prozac were due to the underlying illness of a mood disorder and not because of the medication. We were, to be blunt, reluctant to admit the danger.

Not to be deterred from the pursuit of depression-curing drugs by these warnings, other drug companies developed more SSRIs in rapid succession, including Zoloft, Paxil, Celexa, and Lexapro.

Suicides associated with Prozac use led to court trials.

The tide of public opinion could not be held back indefinitely. In October of 2004, the FDA issued an order that all antidepressants, including Prozac, must carry the government's strongest safety alert, a "black box" warning of the link between the drugs and suicidal thoughts and behavior, especially among children and teenagers. Here is the exact wording of the FDA warning:

FDA Safety Alert for Antidepressants

All pediatrics patients being treated with antidepressants for any indication should be observed closely for clinical worsening, suicidality, and unusual changes in behavior, especially during the initial few months of a course of drug therapy, or at times of dose changes. Observation is defined as one-on-one consultation once a week for the first four weeks of treatment and every other week for the next four weeks with additional visits as warranted.

The latest available evidence indicates that the risk of suicide increases for approximately two percent of persons taking SSRIs. For these persons, the impulse occurs soon after taking the medication and often follows a period of intense agitation.

Each of these drugs has a fascinating history wrapped in competitive zeal and a good dose of advertising hype.

Antidepressants (SSRIs)

Relative Adverse-Effect Profiles

Agent	Usual Adult Dosage (mg/d)	Drowsiness	Sexual Dys-function	Agitation/ Insomnia
Celexa (citalopram)	20-40	moderate	very high	very low
Lexapro (escitalo-pram)	10-20	low	very high	very low
Luvox (fluvoxamine)	100-300	high	very high	low
Paxil (paroxetine)	10-60	moderate	very high	low
Paxil CR	12.5-75	moderate	very high	low
Prozac (fluoxetine)	10-80	low	very high	high
Prozac Weekly	90 mg/wk	low	very high	high
Zoloft (sertraline)	50-200	low	very high	moderate

Adapted from CNS News Special Edition December 2004

From brand name to generic drug

After a patent for a drug is obtained, the developer has a fourteen-year window of exclusive production and marketing. When the patent expires, anyone can produce the drug with the same composition. The drug that is no longer patented is known as a generic drug.

Because they are usually much less expensive than the original product, generic drugs take over a large chunk of the market. This is fine for the retailers selling prescription drugs to the public. Because the markup is much higher for generic drugs than for branded ones, pharmacies have a huge financial incentive to sell them.

Many people do not realize that generic and brand-name drugs are not exactly the same. Generics are required by the FDA to be "bioequivalent" to the original medication, meaning they must mirror the chemical structure and be equally accessible to the body of the person taking them. Almost. The FDA allows a variance of up to twenty percent in the amount of the active ingredient that is absorbed by the body over a specific period of time when approving generics for public use. There are also differences in the coating, binding materials, flavoring and other components, and allergic reactions to these ingredients can be serious.

Pharmaceutical companies sometimes rush to market with new drugs to blunt the competition from generic versions of their own brand products. Some observers believe that the development of the SSRI Lexapro was a marketing ploy by the drug company to shore up sales revenue when Celexa's patent expired.

Differences in SSRIs

We may not understand military strategy, but at least we know that SSRIs are alike in the way they battle depression, right?

Not true. There are significant differences. Paxil, Luvox, and Celexa, for example, tend to have more of a sedating effect on patients, while Prozac, Zoloft and Lexapro may be more stimulating.

When it comes to SSRIs, thinking like a psychiatrist means not being surprised when people respond in quite different ways to a course of treatment utilizing these drugs. The psychiatrist is fully aware of the fact that neither the presence nor the intensity of unintended consequences associated with SSRIs can be predicted accurately from one patient to another.

Discontinuation

Patients experience discomfort when they stop taking SSRIs. Reports of dizziness, nausea, a sensation of being pricked by "pins and needles," and a feeling of being zapped by electricity are fairly common symptoms following abruptly stopping an SSRI.

This problem is least likely to happen with Prozac or Prozac Weekly because it leaves the body more slowly than the other SSRIs. In our experience, abruptly stopping the use of Paxil creates the most dramatic problems.

The reality is that many persons simply do not respond at all to these medications, and for others there will be only a partial response.

Stereochemistry and Prozac's successors

Chemistry students are often baffled when they learn complicated formulas only to discover that two substances with exactly the same molecular formula are actually different compounds. These compounds are known as isomers ("iso" meaning "same"). The best illustration of isometry is to look at your hands. One is the reverse of the other, but your right and left hands have quite different functions.

Stereochemistry: mirror images, like your left and right hands.

Now imagine two molecules that are mirror images of each other. Looking at the spatial arrangement of the compounds we might observe that a plane of light beamed into one of them always rotates to the left, and into the other one always to the right. The designation "S" for "sinister" represents a left rotating action, and an "R" for "rectus" represents action turning toward the right.

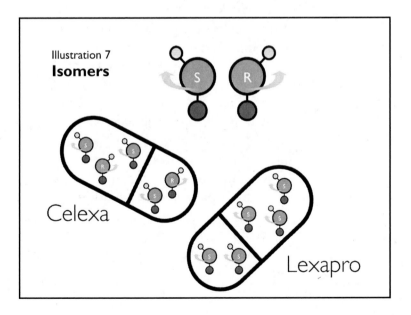

Illustration 7
Isomers

Celexa

Lexapro

An example of mirror images in chemistry is carvon, a chemical found in the oils of many fruits and seeds. It has two versions that are an exact reverse of each other. R-carvon is responsible for the flavor and odor of spearmint, while its mirror image, L-carvon, triggers the taste and smell of caraway seeds. Another example of a stereoisomeric chemical is limonine. R-limonine and L-limonine are responsible for the smell of oranges and lemons, respectively.

Isomers in medications can have quite different effects. Darvon and Novrad (Darvon spelled backwards) are examples. Darvon relieves pain while Novrad is used to control coughing. One isomer can be helpful while the mirror image of the same drug can be toxic. L-dopa, for example, is used to treat symptoms of Parkinson's Disease while its isomer, d-dopa, is toxic.

Most drugs are a mixture of left rotating and right rotating molecules.

Celexa, the trademarked name of an SSRI that has made great strides in replacing Prozac in the market for antidepressants, is a combination of two isomers. Celexa is made from the chemical citalopram, which consists of equal amounts of its R- and S- isomers. This distinction earns Celexa the designation of a "racemate" in the rush to success.

Celexa originated in Europe where it is known as Cipramil but is branded and sold in the U.S. by Forest Laboratories. Its manufacturer, H. Lundbeck, claimed that Celexa delivers more serotonin to brain cells than Prozac and other SSRIs. Sales were brisk, but just as the original patent on Celexa was expiring, the company introduced another SSRI, Lexapro, and claimed it was a better choice. Criticism of manufacturers' claims have cast shadows on its superiority over Celexa. The jury is still out, but many psychiatrists now use Lexapro as their preferred antidepressant.

SNRIs

Next in the "alphabet soup" of psychotropic medicines are the SNRIs, serotonin plus norepinephrine reuptake inhibitors. The "N" represents norepinephrine.

The mechanism is the same as with SSRIs except that this family of drugs interferes with the return of norepinephrine as well as serotonin to the presynaptic neuron. This leaves more of the chemical working on the receptor cells and increases the possibility of positive effects.

In 1993 Wyeth-Ayerst Laboratories introduced the first SNRI as Effexor IR (venlafaxine), an antidepressant that promised to avoid some of the side effects of the SSRIs while delivering all of the benefits. Four years later Wyeth-Ayerst introduced a sustained release medicine, Effexor XR. The newer drug, as promised, had even fewer side effects, and only one pill a day was sufficient to deliver maximum benefits.

Effexor was the first SNRI to be marketed in the U.S.

Cymbalta (duloxetine), released in the summer of 2004, works on the serotonin and norepinephrine neurotransmitters and has been approved for treatment of depression as well as diabetic peripheral neuropathic pain.

SNRIs are approved by the FDA for the treatment of major depressive disorder and general anxiety disorder. Other possible uses are in the treatment of obsessive compulsive disorders, panic disorders, attention deficit hyperactivity disorder (ADHD), fibromyalgia, and chronic pain.

Just as with SSRIs, the potential for a higher risk of suicide in patients taking SNRIs remains a question in determining their future. There is no question, however, that even this medication class has side effects (nausea, sleepiness or insomnia, dizziness, nervousness, increased blood pressure). Problems when the drug is discontinued can be even worse than those encountered with SSRIs.

Wellbutrin

The antidepressant Wellbutrin has lived a turbulent existence in the psychopharmaceutical market. GlaxoSmith-Kline, a pharmaceutical company based in the United Kingdom, invented an antidepressant with the chemical name bupropion HCL in 1966 when GlaxoSmithKline was the Burroughs-Wellcome company. The name, "Wellbutrin," is a combination of "Wellcome" and "bupropion."

Although Wellbutrin was approved in 1985 by the FDA as an antidepressant, the drug was pulled off the market when clinical trials found that seizures were occurring

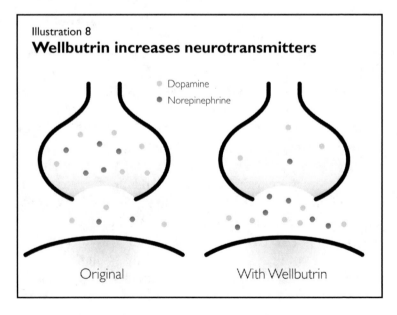

Illustration 8
Wellbutrin increases neurotransmitters

Dopamine
Norepinephrine

Original

With Wellbutrin

two to four times more often in patients taking Wellbutrin than in those taking other antidepressants.

After further research, Wellbutrin was re-released with a warning not to prescribe for patients with a history of bulimia or a chance of seizures. Its arrival was heralded with great enthusiasm as the first antidepressant without any sexual side effects.

Twelve years later Wellbutrin was approved by the FDA as an aid to breaking the nicotine habit and was sold in the U.S. as Zyban.

Wellbutrin comes in three "flavors:" IR (immediate release), taken three times a day; SR (sustained release), taken two times a day; and XL (extended release) taken once a day. Today we can obtain bupropion as Zyban or Wellbutrin, or as generic bupropion. As an antidepressant, Wellbutrin is advertised as unique because it acts directly on the nerve cells rather than on the reuptake mechanism that is the focus of SSRIs and SNRIs. Wellbutrin works by enhancing the release of norepinephrine and dopamine. The FDA has approved of Wellbutrin in the treatment of depression. Off-label uses include treating attention deficit hyperactivity disorder (ADHD) and obesity as well as in counteracting the sexual side effects of SSRIs.

There is still, however, an increased risk of seizures by patients taking Wellbutrin, and if you or someone you are caring for is using Wellbutrin, you should be aware of this. Of course you know that seizures are much more likely in individuals who suffer from seizure disorders or eating disorders—or have experienced a head injury in the past.

Other side effects observed include anxiety, agitation, insomnia, nausea, tremor, and weight loss.

Other antidepressants

Antidepressants deserving a brief summary in this discussion include Remeron (mirtazapine), Desyrel (trazodone), and Serzone (nefazodone).

The drug company Organon, Inc., received FDA approval of Remeron to treat depression in 1996. Remeron increases the amount of serotonin and norepinephrine in brain cells but not by utilizing the reuptake mechanism used by SSRIs or SNRIs.

Off-label uses for Remeron include inducing sleep and relieving severe anxiety.

Many patients taking Remeron gain a few pounds. Some patients become incredibly hungry and gain a significant amount of weight. Actually, this can be useful in malnourished patients, proving the point that not every side effect is negative. It depends on the individual patient.

Remeron is often used in combination with other medicines in treatment-resistant depression. The sedative action of the drug can result in excessive sleepiness. "I slept for three days," was a common comment about Remeron's most common side effect. Studies were done looking at using Remeron to treat sleep disorders, but that project has been cancelled.

"I slept for three days"—comment by many Remeron users.

Desyrel is approved as an antidepressant in the U.S. Desyrel is not a reuptake inhibitor but increases the availability of serotonin in the brain. As a psychiatrist, I view this medicine more as a sleeping pill than an antidepressant. Most patients cannot tolerate the sedation that accompanies doses required to treat depression.

Patients who like Desyrel say it helps them enjoy restful, calm sleep at night. However, they may continue to feel sleepy into the next day. A potentially dangerous side effect that occurs rarely with Desyrel is a condition called priapism, the prolonged erection of the penis without sexual stimulation. Blood doesn't drain from the penis, causing pain and risking permanent damage to the penis without immediate treatment.

Serzone was never a popular antidepressant, although it had fewer side effects than Desyrel. The brand name was withdrawn from the U.S. market in 2004 due to potentially fatal liver problems associated

> **Treating depression is NOT a chemical balancing act.**

with its use and disappointing sales. The generic version of Serzone, nefazodone, is still available.

The future of antidepressants

Be sure not to fall into the trap of believing that the key to a depression-free life is "chemical balance." When you take aspirin to relieve a headache, you are not correcting an aspirin deficiency. In the same way, the mechanism of antidepressant medications is more intricate than simply boosting levels of certain chemicals to achieve balance. The medications that treat depression do much more.

We are seeing a growing body of evidence showing that individual response to antidepressants not only includes short-term changes in chemical balance but also brings about long-term structural changes to the brain.

You may have heard that we are born with a definite number of brain cells and that we can't make new ones. This is a myth. Throughout our lifetimes all of us make new neurons in a specialized area of our brain called the hippocampus. People under stress make fewer new neurons, a big risk factor for depression. The hippocampus of a person who has been chronically depressed may be 20 percent smaller than that of a non-depressed person.

The good news is that taking an antidepressant for at least a few weeks can increase neurogenesis, the creation of new neurons.

Scientists believe that the increased formation of neurons is one of many possible ways that antidepressants work. We now have evidence that the presence of more neurons and the new connections between them enhances communications. Scientists refer to the way that antidepressants change the number and sensitivity of receptors in the brain as "downregulation."

You can read an excellent explanation for the way neurons are formed in the hippocampus in an article by L. Santarelli *et al* in the August 8, 2003, edition of *Science* (pages 805-809).

Changes in the way neurotransmitters are balanced in the brain begin within a few hours of taking an antidepressant, but it can take weeks or months for a clinical response. This is why patience is required while waiting for the results we seek. Antidepressants do not work immediately.

Antidepressants do not take effect right away.

We will see more sophistication in the development of antidepressants. Even more promising, I believe, will be new discoveries in the use of peptides and hormones to deal with the intricate and complex chemical reactions in our brains.

Much of the depression we suffer in the U.S. today is a result of stress. I believe that in the next decade we will find new and effective medicines to help people reduce levels of harmful stress so they can cope with stress that cannot be avoided.

Antidepressants in development

By the time this book has been printed and distributed, more antidepressants will probably be in general use. Following is updated information about antidepressants under development in 2007.

Gepirone ER. Gepirone ER is currently in clinical trials and thus far looks promising for patients with major depression. This new medication represents the first in a new class of antidepressants, the direct serotonin agonists. Officially, gepirone is known as a 5-HT1, a partial agonist. This medication could provide a new treatment possibility for patients who didn't have success with current available treatments.

The side effects of gepirone are few: transient light-headedness, headache, and nausea. The good news is that other side effects that usually occur with antidepressant treatment, such as sexual dysfunction, were not seen in any patients involved in any of their studies. We will see!

Valdoxan (agomelatine). Valdoxan is the first melaton-ergic (MT1 and MT2 receptor) agonist antidepressant and has several potential advantages over existing treatments. [See Rozerem on page 116 for more information about melatonin receptors.] Besides being an effective antidepressant, Valdoxan has shown particular advantages in improving disrupted sleep patterns of depressed patients without affecting daytime vigilance. Valdoxan is the only antidepressant with specific action on circadian rhythms, which are often imbalanced in depressed patients.

In a study over eight weeks, Valdoxan was shown to be an effective antidepressant at a dose of 25 milligram once daily in adults of all ages, including the severely depressed and elderly depressed. In this study there were no signs of discontinuation symptoms, and, unlike many antidepressants, it does not appear to impair sexual function or cause weight gain.

Valdoxan may be coming to Europe within the next year. Hopefully, we will see it in the United States shortly after.

DVS-233 SR. Wyeth, the manufacturer of DVS-233 SR (desvenlafaxine) is currently awaiting an approval decision from the FDA for the active metabolite of Effexor (venlafaxine). Whether the development of this drug is a way to extend patient life as Effexor goes generic or whether it will offer added benefits over Effexor remains to be seen. Trials have been completed not only for depression but also for the treatment of moderate to severe vasomotor symptoms (such as hot flashes and night sweats) associated with menopause.

Reboxetine. The introduction of reboxetine (or an isomer) in the U.S. is almost inevitable. Available in twenty-two countries around the world, this antidepressant binds to the norepinephrine transportation molecule to block its reuptake. Because this drug does not affect serotonin, the side effects are different. Especially valuable in this regard is a decreased likelihood of sexual side effects resulting from its use.

A preliminary letter of approval was granted by the FDA in 1999, but trials conducted in the U.S. and Canada resulted in another letter of non-approval, and the status of the drug's approval in the U.S. as of this writing is uncertain.

Ixel (milnacipran). Another SNRI, Ixel is being developed as a successor to Effexor and Cymbalta. This drug may be approved by the FDA for treatment of depression and fibromyalgia. It has already been approved in 22 countries for the treatment of depression.

Vilazadone. In early clinical trials in late 2004, the chemical compound vilazodone proved effective in the treatment of depression with minimal side effects. Vilazodone relies on a dual mechanism involving SSRI as well as a specific serotonin receptor called 5HT1A to affect serotonin in two ways. Genetic testing could play a role in determining the best use of this drug.

Nemifitide. A synthetic brain peptide antidepressant, Nemfitide is being tested as a powerful new therapeutic tool in the treatment of depression. This medicine is given by a series of injections that may be given as infrequently as once in four to six months. It appears in early studies to have an earlier and more robust onset of action—as early as three to five days.

Preliminary results of a large trial involving more than 400 patients are expected by mid 2007.

Corlux. Originally known as RU-486, the abortion pill, Corlux is an antagonist of one of the body's two cortisol receptors and its progesterone receptor. A receptor antagonist is a molecule that stops the normal function of a receptor. Corlux is potentially effective in treating psychotic depression.

Studies in psychiatry involving Corlux were implemented to determine its ability to treat psychotic depression. So far it has been shown to be well tolerated, and can also be taken with other antipsychotic or antidepressant medications without complications.

The most attractive characteristic of Corlux that makes it a desirable choice to treat severe depression is that it works very quickly, with patients seeing significant relief within seven days after the treatment has begun. Psychiatrists at Stanford are still doing research on this application of Corlux and despite a recent negative trial, remain positive about its potential benefits to those most severely ill.

CRF antagonists. Corticotropin releasing factor-1 (CRF) receptor antagonists are currently in development to treat not only depression but anxiety as well. CRF functions as a neurotransmitter in the brain and plays a critical role in coordinating the body's response to stress. The CRF-1 receptor subtype largely mediates these effects. In animal models, selective CRF-1 receptor antagonists block stress-related responses which may result in improved antianxiety and antidepressant properties. Some data suggest that CRF-1 antagonists may have a more rapid onset of action and a better side effect profile compared to currently marketed antidepressants.

SR 58611. This drug, by Sanofi-Aventis, is a beta-3-adrenoceptor agonist originally pursued as a potential treatment for irritable bowel syndrome and obesity but is now in development for depression. Blocking these beta adrenergic receptors has been associated with mood downturn and depression, presumably because turning on these beta receptors stimulates the production and release of important neurotransmitters such as norepinephrine and serotonin. (See information about beta blockers such as Inderal on page 45) The selectivity of SR 58611 for the beta-3 receptor is high, in the hopes of producing an antidepressant effect without producing other cardiac or respiratory side effects.

Other possibilities. Sanofi also is exploring Saredutant (SR 48968), a NK2 antagonist. Pfizer is studying another

NK variant. CP-122721 is a neurokinin 1 (NK-1) antagonist being developed as a possible treatment for depression and inflammatory diseases including asthma and irritable bowel syndrome. Roche has R673, another NK-1 receptor antagonist in development. GW 597599 is a neurokinin-1 (NK-1) receptor antagonist. It is currently in phase II trials by GSK for chemotherapy-induced vomiting, depression and anxiety. I told you that peptides were hot!

And so are hormones. GlaxoSmithKline (GSK) and Neurocrine Biosciences are investigating a series of corticotropin releasing factor-1 (CRF-1) receptor antagonists, for the treatment of various neurological and gastrointestinal disorders including anxiety and depression.

LuAA21004 is a serotonin modulator and stimulator that belongs to a psychotropic class of chemical compounds known as bis-aryl-sulphanyl amines. This medication has a new pharmacological profile combining serotonin reuptake inhibition with a number of other characteristics, including activation of monoaminergic systems. It is under investigation by Lundbeck for the treatment of depression.

DOV-21947 is a triple reuptake inhibitor under investigation by DOV Pharmaceuticals for the treatment of depression. The term "triple reuptake inhibitor" means it blocks the reuptake of serotonin and norepinephrine (like Effexor) with the bonus of also blocking the reuptake of dopamine. Results of extensive testing are expected soon.

Antianxiety Agents

Anxiety disorders cover a wide range of problems. Examples of anxiety include panic attacks, obsessive compulsive disorder, post-traumatic stress disorder, and generalized anxiety. Phobias are a common form of anxiety marked by irrational fear of height, crowds, or other situations that are not in themselves threatening.

Medications to lessen the symptoms of anxiety have been developed over the past few decades, and many of them are highly effective.

Just as with depression, the primary goal of the psychiatrist in treating anxiety is full remission—the elimination of all symptoms. Anxiety is so tenacious that this goal is seldom reached, but failure to act decisively and early when serious symptoms of anxiety surface can be disastrous.

The short-term goal in treating anxiety disorders is to stop the anxiety before it becomes uncontrollable. In the long term, the goal is to prevent such attacks from occurring.

Anxiety can progress rapidly even as the patient does everything possible to avoid recurrences. Once victimized by anxiety, the person is literally terrified of the possibility of another episode. He or she may avoid every situation similar to the one that triggered the last attack. The situation can progress to the point of total withdrawal or agoraphobia, the medical term for a fear of the marketplace, crowds, and every aspect of life outside the person's immediate environment.

I remember my first trip across the San Mateo Bridge near San Francisco. Coming from the Midwest where roads are straight and the landscape is even, I found that the idea of manipulating my car across a weaving ribbon of concrete above the ocean was too much for me. There is no stopping once you're on that bridge, and if you slow down you risk the wrath of every other driver behind you, not to mention the crunch of metal on metal if you swerve out of your lane or, worse, the horrid splash into the water. Add to that the awful sensation of the swaying back and forth of that huge structure, and the effect on me of driving on the bridge was horrific.

I made it across that first time, shaking and trembling all the way. Later, when I learned there was another way of getting to the other side of the bay without taking the bridge, I gladly drove an extra eighty miles to avoid another terrifying experience.

Full relief from an anxiety disorder is rare.

Eventually I overcame my initial fear of the bridge and did not require a course of psychotropic medication to return me to a normal mind-set. Others are not that fortunate.

By far the hardest variety of these problems to treat effectively is the obsessive compulsive disorder, abbreviated as OCD. Those of us not directly affected by OCD are amused by the idea of being driven to repeat a useless activity over and over. For the person so afflicted, OCD is no laughing matter.

Many options are available to the psychiatrist to determine the cause and extent of an anxiety order. Both short-term and long-term needs of the patient must be considered in choosing the most effective option for each patient. This is not always easy, since anxiety disorders differ from each other in significant ways. Even if the symptoms can be accurately defined, people respond differently to the same medication or treatment course. This is what makes psychiatry such an invigorating challenge.

Drug therapy may be thwarted by the patient's resistance to the prescribed medication. Anxious patients are particularly sensitive to side effects. The long list of potential problems the druggist hands the patient who has come to get a prescription filled will only add to the person's anxiety. Too often, patients with anxiety disorders simply do not want to take medications for their problem. The patient may refuse to follow the doctor's orders or may comply halfheartedly. For these reasons the therapist needs to see the patient frequently enough during the early phases of treatment to evaluate how the patient is responding and, more importantly, to provide reassurance and education.

A willing patient is a treatable patient.

A willing patient is a treatable patient, and information and trust are the keys to a positive patient-therapist relationship.

How do antianxiety agents work?

Just as with depression, antianxiety agents do not "cure" anxiety or guarantee that the person will never experience anxiety again. They are effective in blunting the symptoms of anxiety so that the individual can resume normal activities.

Antianxiety pharmaceutical agents, or anxiolytics, work primarily on serotonin and GABA neurotransmitters.

As we have seen, antidepressants are agents that work on serotonin and other neurotransmitters, so it should be no surprise to learn that antidepressants are also effective in treating anxiety disorders. With the exception of Wellbutrin, antidepressants also have a good likelihood for reducing the symptoms of anxiety.

The antidepressants used most often to treat anxiety include Zoloft, Paxil, Celexa and Lexapro, and Effexor XR.

The biggest drawback in relying on these medications is that they may not make a difference for weeks, and by definition, anxiety is a time-sensitive condition. Obviously, antidepressants are not good tools for stopping a panic attack.

Another problem with using antidepressants to treat anxiety is that side effects may actually worsen anxiety at first. Imagine the impact on an already anxious and fearful person when increased stomach distress, tremors, and problems sleeping follow their use of antidepressants.

Overall, the most promising use of antidepressants in treating anxiety is to help prevent future anxiety attacks.

Benzodiazepines

The granddaddy of benzodiazepines, Valium (diazepam), was once the most prescribed medicine in the world. Unfortunately, Valium has also been identified as habit forming. Other benzodiazepines include Xanax (alprazolam), Ativan (lorazepam), Klonopin (clonazepam), and many others.

Valium—the granddaddy of all the benzos.

The FDA has approved these medications for the treatment of a variety of anxiety-related problems. The list varies from drug to drug but may include anxiety, panic, alcohol withdrawal, muscle spasms, seizures, insomnia, uncontrolled periodic limb movement, and neuralgia.

Anxiolytics (Benzodiazepines)

Pharmacokinetic Parameters

Agent	Approved Indications	Approved Oral Adult Dosage Range (mg/d	Onset (PO)	t½
Ativan (lorazepam)	Anxiety; preoperative sedation	1-8 / 1-4 mg single dose	fast	short
Klonopin (clonazepam)	seizure disorders; panic disorder	0.5-2	moderate	long
Librium (chlordiazep-oxide)	anxiety, alcohol withdrawal; preoperative sedation	5-100 / 25-50 mg single dose	fast	long
Serax (oxazepam)	anxiety disorders; alcohol withdrawal	30-120	slow	short
Tranxene (clorazepate)	anxiety, seizure disorders; alcohol withdrawal	15-60	very fast	long
Valium (diazepam)	anxiety, alcohol withdrawal; muscle spasm; preoperative sedation; status epilepticus	2-40 / 2-10 mg single dose	very fast	long
Xanax (alprazolam)	Anxiety disorders; panic disorder	0.25-04	fast	inter-mediate

Adapted from CNS News Special Edition December 2004

The most dangerous risk of taking benzodiazepines is the potential for getting caught in its addictive grip. The drugs take effect immediately, giving a good feeling. Tolerance may quickly build so that stronger doses are needed to achieve the same level of well-being. When the drug is discontinued, withdrawal symptoms including seizures can occur.

Film makers have seized on this danger with movies such as "I am Dancing as Fast as I Can." Realistically, the risk of addiction is actually quite small.

Side effects other than addiction can also be dangerous. Besides feeling sedated, a person taking benzodiazepines may experience ataxia (loss of balance) and slurred speech. An elderly person could fall and be seriously injured as a result. Impaired memory may also occur as an additional unwanted side effect.

How benzodiazepines work

All of these medications work on the principle that an anxiety circuit in the brain causes the emotional response we call anxiety. By blocking the circuit, the medication prevents anxiety from occurring; instead, the person taking the medication feels calm and peaceful. If this sounds to you like the mellow feeling you experience after drinking alcoholic beverages, you have correctly identified alcohol as another chemical that uses the same mechanism to disable the anxiety circuit.

Buspirone differs from other anxiety drugs

Another antianxiety agent we'll consider is BuSpar (buspirone), a medication that is not related in either a chemical or a pharmaceutical sense to benzodiazepines or other anti-anxiety agents.

BuSpar works both presynaptically and postsynaptically to modulate the effects of serotonin on receptors. In other words, buspirone is able to normalize the production of serotonin. In Illustration 9 you can see buspirone working to regulate serotonin on both sides of the synapse.

BuSpar is approved by the FDA for the treatment of anxiety and is also prescribed off label to deal with excessive agitation, especially among the elderly.

The mental health community had high hopes for BuSpar because it promised to treat anxiety without the negatives of drugs like Valium. After several years on the market, however, BuSpar lost its aura and is now seen as ineffective by many practitioners.

The main issue with BuSpar is that it does not work immediately like benzos. It can take weeks to become effective, so if patients want instant relief, they won't get it from BuSpar. Besides the fact that BuSpar's benefits occur later than with benzodiazepines, regular use of the drug is associated with side effects such as sedation, dizziness, nausea, and headache.

BuSpar can take weeks to become effective.

The usual strategy for dealing with people who are suffering from anxiety attacks is to combine benzodiazepine with an antidepressant in the early stage of treatment and then taper off the "benzo" after the effect of the antidepressants kicks in.

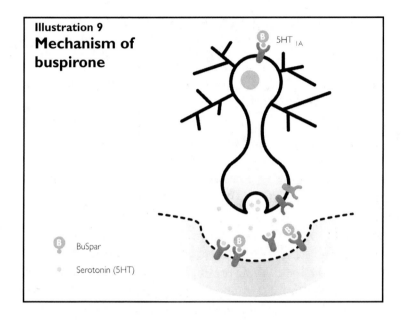

Illustration 9
Mechanism of buspirone

5HT$_{1A}$

B BuSpar

· Serotonin (5HT)

New developments in antianxiety medications

PRX-00023 is a serotonin-1A (5HT$_{1a}$) receptor agonist similar to buspirone. Unlike the older medicine, it does not need to be taken several times daily. It is under investigation by Predix Pharmaceuticals for the treatment of generalized anxiety disorder (GAD) and depression. So far, the most common side effect in clinical trials is flu-like symptoms.

MN-305 is a selective serotonin 5HT$_{1a}$ receptor agonist under investigation by MediciNova for the treatment of anxiety and depression as well as for additional neurological indications including the treatment of jet-lag syndrome. Results from animal studies showed that the drug suppressed psychological stress-induced elevations of dopamine and serotonin.

Antipsychotics

Probably the most challenging of all mental disorders is psychosis because it is both serious and persistent—and it eludes effective treatment.

"Psychosis," one of my patients told me, "makes you feel an amazing amount of fear."

Psychiatrists know from the first day that they are unlikely to achieve a result even close to full remission. The goal is to identify and treat the disease as soon as possible in order to stop it in its tracks and prevent it from overcoming the person. Management, not healing, is the operative word for treating persons diagnosed with psychotic disorders. Patients may have good reasons to refuse medication, and they deserve the best support available to be sure they are tracking well with their treatment plan.

A person with psychosis usually realizes that something is terribly wrong.

Psychotic persons have insight. They know something is drastically wrong. "My mind was like a burned-out field," a patient being treated for psychosis said to me. "I felt totally barren, that my mind had been destroyed."

After being successfully treated for symptoms of psychosis, he started piecing together what had happened. "It took a combination of drugs to bring me back," he said. In his case a careful combination of Depakote, Risperdal, and Anafranil helped him deal effectively with symptoms of OCD and depression as well as psychosis.

The mantra of medical practice—to do no harm—must be followed studiously by the professional psychiatrist and other persons providing care or emotional support to these individuals.

Development of antipsychotic agents

For a historical perspective of antipsychotic therapy in the U.S., consider the following chart showing the development of four drugs between 1950 and 1965 that were reasonably successful followed by a twenty-year hiatus in antipsychotic drug research and development.

The first drugs approved for psychotic disorders are now called "conventional" or "typical." Drugs in this category developed after 1985 are called "atypical." Specifically, atypical antipsychotics involved other receptors and proved to be more effective in treating symptoms of schizophrenia with fewer neurologic and other side effects.

Leading the race with conventional drugs to treat psychotic disorders effectively was Thorazine (chlorpromazine). It was reported as successful in treating schizophrenia in 1952. In its path, other drugs with a similar chemical structure were developed. These included Trilafon (perphenazine) and Prolixin (fluphenazine), followed by compounds such as Mellaril (thioridazine), Haldol (haloperidol) and Orap (pimozide) with different chemical structures.

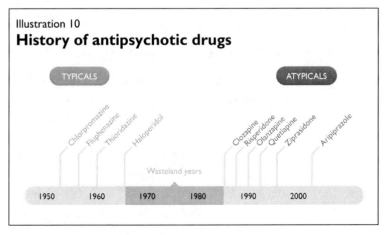

Illustration 10
History of antipsychotic drugs

The first atypical antipsychotic agent on the scene was Clozaril (clozapine), approved by the FDA in 1990 to treat patients with schizophrenia that had resisted previous methods of treatment. Its main benefit was that fewer patients taking the drug experienced the frustration known as EPS or extrapyramidal syndrome, a condition that can range from a general state of restlessness to muscular spasms of the neck, eyes, tongue, or jaw, and drug-induced Parkinson disease. It also appeared to be more potent and effective than any antipsychotic before it.

Newer antipsychotics include Risperdal (risperidone), Zyprexa (olanzapine), Seroquel (quetiapine), Geodon (ziprasidone), and Abilify (aripiprazole).

Antipsychotic medications are powerful and carry with them the risk of serious side effects. Earlier medications in this category were associated with a variety of negative effects, including over sedation, breathing disorders, tremor, rigidity, repetitive muscle movement, seizures, and weight gains.

The newer, or atypical, antipsychotic agents generally produce better results with fewer side effects. As a result, patients are more likely to comply with the doctor's prescription for them.

Choosing an antipsychotic agent

When you think like a psychiatrist, you are faced with a panel of choices. You must decide on a treatment that will be effective in lessening the symptoms of schizophrenia without causing weight gain, diabetes, sexual dysfunction, heart problems or other serious side effects. The combination of effective relief from symptoms with few drawbacks is a recipe for success in any plan to treat mental disorders.

Most antipsychotic medications are prescribed by psychiatrists, but private care providers account for up to thirty percent of prescriptions for drugs in this category.

How antipsychotic medications work

All antipsychotics work on dopamine and serotonin; some involve other neurotransmitters as well.

The theory behind psychotic disorders such as schizophrenia is that in affected individuals, excess dopamine is released from the mesolimbic pathway and postsynaptic receptors are overstimulated. This leads to the development of symptoms such as hallucinations.

In patients with schizophrenia, too little dopamine is released within the mesocortical pathway, and the postsynaptic receptors are understimulated. This hypoactivity is thought to cause negative symptoms such as lack of motivation and apathy.

The older psychotic agents tended to block dopamine from all pathways, so that psychotic symptoms were improved, but the areas of the brain that needed dopamine were punished. Severe problems such as lactation and other negative symptoms occurred. Extrapyramidal symptoms (EPS) are experienced by up to 60 percent of persons taking typical psychotic drugs such as Haldol.

Remember that dopamine is the "pleasure chemical" (see page 39). It is also responsible for motivation, concentration, and energy.

A person with too much dopamine may have what we call "positive symptoms" of psychosis, which are not positive in the sense of being good. Hallucinations, delusions, and confused thinking are examples of occurrences that are

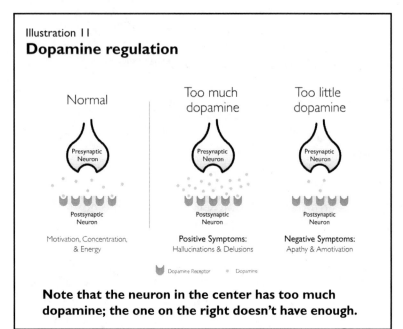

Illustration 11
Dopamine regulation

Normal	Too much dopamine	Too little dopamine
Presynaptic Neuron	Presynaptic Neuron	Presynaptic Neuron
Postsynaptic Neuron	Postsynaptic Neuron	Postsynaptic Neuron
Motivation, Concentration, & Energy	Positive Symptoms: Hallucinations & Delusions	Negative Symptoms: Apathy & Amotivation

Dopamine Receptor   Dopamine

Note that the neuron in the center has too much dopamine; the one on the right doesn't have enough.

beyond normal experience and therefore, in medical terminology, "positive."

By contrast, not having enough dopamine leads to "negative" symptoms such as apathy and lack of motivation. They are called negative symptoms of psychosis because they imply a diminished experience. The objective of antipsychotic medications is to regulate the amount of dopamine in the parts of the brain that need it and leave the rest alone.

Antipsychotics have been approved by the FDA for treatment of psychosis, schizophrenia, bipolar mania, nausea and vomiting, Tourette's syndrome, and chronic hiccups. Off-label uses may include treatment of a variety of conditions, including extreme agitation, behavioral problems, Alzheimer disease, insomnia, and depression.

Newer antipsychotic agents

The first atypical antipsychotic drug to be approved by the FDA was Clozaril. The use of this drug is statistically linked to a higher risk of diabetes, weight gain, low or nonexistent production of white blood cells to fight infections (agranulocytosis), and heart complications. Because of the risk of agranulocytosis, weekly blood tests are required by patients taking Clozaril for the first six months of treatment followed by bi-weekly tests as long as the person is taking the medication. This adds significantly to the cost of treatment.

The FDA has warned the medical profession of the possibility of these adverse reactions, and warnings for the patient to read are now packaged with the pills.

The second of the newer generation of antipsychosis agents to be developed was Risperdal. This drug has the embarrassing but not life-threatening effect of increasing prolactin levels in the brain. Prolactin is the brain hormone that signals the human breasts to manufacture milk, and it can affect men, women, or children.

On the positive side, Risperdal has a long history of safety, is less expensive, and is associated with less weight gain than some of the other antipsychotic drugs.

Prolactin can stimulate milk production, even in men.

Zyprexa was approved by the FDA in 1996 for the long-term treatment of persons with schizophrenia as well as other psychotic states and has been prescribed for more than 14 million people since then. Weight gain, risk of diabetes, and unwanted sedation are the main side effects associated with this drug. One 20 milligram pill per day would cost about $640 per month, placing Zyprexa in the "expensive" category.

At least one patient is furious with Eli Lilly for its advertising program for Zyprexa. A 52-year-old man in

Indiana sued the drug company for false claims about the drug's effectiveness in treating depression. Many other lawsuits have been launched claiming that Zyprexa led to diabetes in patients being treated with the drug for symptoms of schizophrenia. Before the storm ended, more than 8,000 people had filed lawsuits for developing diabetes and other diseases after taking Zyprexa. The final settlement cost the company more than $250 million for payments, legal fees, and associated costs. The average amount awarded to patients was $50,000.

Seroquel is another atypical antipsychotic medication that does not seem to cause many of the side effects that made the earlier drugs in this category undesirable, such as tardive dyskinesia, and seizures. It is, however, associated with weight gain to some degree, and it may be overly sedating for some persons.

> **Geodon met with a cold reception, then passed trials with flying colors.**

When Geodon came on the scene in 1998 as a promising new drug combatting symptoms of schizophrenia, it met with a cold reception. At first the FDA was concerned about the possibility of increased risk of fatal irregularities in heartbeat. Specifically, evidence indicated that the portion of the heartbeat known as the QT interval was often longer than normal in persons taking the drug. This condition can lead to dangerous irregularities in heart rhythms.

Three years later, after re-evaluating safety data, the FDA in 2001 approved Geodon for treating schizophrenia. In the side effects department, Geodon passed clinical trials with flying colors. Large clinical trials showed minimal connection between the drug and weight gain, the most common side effect associated with similar medications.

Abilify was approved by the FDA in 2002 as the latest in the atypical group of medications offering hope to persons suffering from schizophrenia. The new drug is effective without long delays, promises no problems with the QT interval in the heartbeat, results in minimal weight gain, and delivers highly effective results with one pill per day taken with or without food. Side effects are uncommon but may include a condition of internal restlessness known as akathisia as well as either insomnia or drowsiness—opposite conditions that can be triggered in different persons by the same agent.

Ampakines, abbreviated as AMPA, are small benzamide compounds that modulate receptors to produce positive performance on behavioral tasks. According to early research, ampakine compounds enhance glutamate pathways, which interact with dopamine and serotonin systems in order to maintain normal brain function. The glutamate pathways are believed to be depressed in patients with schizophrenia, contributing to problems in memory, cognition and attention. This could start a whole new way of treating schizophrenia.

Side effects of antipsychotic medications

Side effects have always been a concern in prescribing and using antipsychotic medications.

Among the conventional antipsychotics, the most worrisome side effect is tardive dyskinesia. (The word "tardive" means "late," and "dyskinesia" means "movement disorder.") A person with this condition twitches or engages in other meaningless motions such as smacking the lips, sticking the tongue out, blinking eyes rapidly, or grimacing. You might come across the resident of a home for the aged dancing in the aisles. This behavior is probably due to an undesirable effect of the medication and not to any improvement in the person's underlying mental state.

Every year approximately five percent of persons treated with conventional antipsychotics are afflicted with tardive dyskinesia, often—but not always—delayed until months after the person starts taking the offending medication. There is no cure for tardive dyskinesia, which often becomes a permanent condition.

For the newer, atypical, antipsychotic agents, the main side effect is an increased risk of Type II diabetes. Research is under way to determine which of the newer drugs have less risk of causing this severe medical problem. Some believe that diabetes is associated with the weight gain commonly associated with the class of drugs. Others believe it is due to underlying psychotic illness.

The risk of Type II diabetes is higher with atypical antipsychotic medicines.

Still others suggest it is directly related to the chemistry of the drug. These issues are under investigation by researchers.

Weight gain is a common side effect of the atypical antipsychotic medications. Other side effects vary according to the specific drug used and may include dry mouth, and constipation. The alarming but treatable condition known as extrapyramidal syndrome (EPS) is associated with the use of Risperdal. See page 91 for more information about EPS.

A major problem with antipsychotic medications is their cost. In California the amount paid to pharmacists for these drugs under MediCal skyrocketed from about $5 million in 1998 to over $40 million four years later, an eightfold increase. During this same time period, the amount paid for antidepressants grew from under $5 million to $15 million.

An antipsychotic drug being developed at this time by Vanda, a small pharmaceutical company, is known as ORG-24448. This drug is based on the action of ampakines, benzamide compounds that modulate AMPA receptors to produce positive performance on behavioral tasks. According to early research, ampakine compounds enhance glutamate pathways, which interact with dopamine and serotonin systems in order to maintain normal brain function. The glutamate pathways are believed to be depressed in patients with schizophrenia, contributing to problems in memory, cognition and attention. This approach could start a whole new way of treating schizophrenia.

Coming soon in the treatment of psychotic disorders may be an implant that will deliver medication in a controlled dose for up to six months.

Mood Stabilizers

All of us have mood swings. One morning we wake up feeling invigorated and ready to chop our way through the jungle of life. The next morning we groan about the prospects of crawling out of bed.

For some persons, these mood swings get in the way of living a normal life. We call the problem of persistent and disruptive mood swings a bipolar disorder. In medical terms the mood swings are labeled "manic" or "depressive."

Many creative people suffer from bipolar disorder and are their most productive selves when their mood is at the extremely high or "manic" state. The German composer Robert Schumann died at the age of 31 after composing more than six hundred songs and dozens of other compositions in a flurry of creativity only to sink into a dark despair up to the time of his death. Some believe he had bipolar disorder.

The oldest substance used to help persons whose mood swings are out of control is lithium, a naturally occurring salt you can buy at the grocery store to replace table salt. The story of lithium and its role in the treatment of mental disorders since its discovery in 1817 deserves a book all its own. Lithium is a chemical element that works like sodium and potassium to create salts. In the brain lithium modifies the way neurotransmitters communicate with nerve cells resulting in a more balanced mix of neurochemicals.

Lithium—salty and helpful in controlling mood swings.

For half a century lithium was used to treat manic-depressive persons before anyone knew what the mechanism might be. In the last century it was suggested that too much of the neurotransmitter glutamate in the synapse between neurons causes mania, and too little results in feelings of depression. One possibility is that lithium keeps levels of active glutamate at a constant level, thus stabilizing the person's moods. We still do not fully understand how lithium works to help achieve emotional balance, but we do know that if carefully managed, a course of treatment involving lithium can be life saving.

Lithium is highly effective, with some studies indicating a success rate of seventy to eighty percent among persons with bipolar disorder. The two leading brand name lithium products are Lithobid and Eskalith. Lithium is also used to treat treatment-resistant depression.

Too much lithium can be lethal, and there is a narrow margin of error between therapeutic and toxic levels of lithium. Monitoring of blood levels is needed at least every three to six months to be sure this doesn't happen.

Anticonvulsants are also prescribed to treat mood swings. Depakote (divalproex) and Lamictal (lamotrigine) are approved by the FDA, and Neurontin (gabapentin), Topamax (topiramate), Tegretol (carbamazepine), and Trileptal (oxcarbazepine), are used off label by many psychiatrists.

Among antipsychotic agents that have been approved by the FDA for use as mood stabilizers are Symbyax (a combination of Prozac and Zyprexa), Seroquel, Risperdal, Abilify, and Geodon.

The goal of mood stabilizers

Continuous relief from the symptoms of bipolar disorder is seldom achieved. Instead, we focus on treating the disorder before it escalates into more serious problems for the individual.

When you think like a psychiatrist, you are aware that the full remission for patients with bipolar disorder is highly unlikely. The goal is to treat the disease quickly so that it doesn't progress. This goal is based on an interesting but unproven theory known as "kindling," the idea that severe mental illness begins with something like an abnormal spark in the brain. We need to treat this event like a spark in the forest and act to stop the fire when it's still just a spark.

The logic is that seizures start small and infrequently, becoming more common and more severe as time goes by. Related to this is the idea that the more episodes of seizures you have, the more you will have in the future.

There is no proof for the validity of these ideas.

The psychiatrist and caregiver have many choices in meeting the short-term and long-term needs of individuals with manic and depressive episodes that interfere with daily life.

Some patients may not want treatment. As frightening as a manic "high" may be, it can be thrilling and invigorating. To some patients the exuberance of the mania is well worth the despair of the down side that inevitably follows. And no illegal drugs are involved. Kay Jamison, a renowned psychologist, describes the ups and downs of her own struggles with bipolar disorder in her book, *An Unquiet Mind.*

The exuberance may be worth the despair.

Neurotransmitters, especially dopamine, serotonin, norepinephrine, and glutamate, create mood abnormalities. The mechanism is not known.

An important point to note is that persons who have bipolar illness are not necessarily psychotic. They can be totally in touch with reality and not suffer from delusions or hallucinations that mark the life of a person with psychosis.

"You have so much energy in the manic state. You're zooming off the wire. I was in high school, and I had clashes with the vice principal all the time. I'd get in confrontations with my teachers almost every minute. I had a foul mouth and spewed out ugly words at every opportunity. Teachers would warn each other that I was coming so they'd be ready to deal with me."

—An adolescent who experienced the "high" of the bipolar disorder

There is no single effective way to approach the treatment of bipolar disorder. Many patients require a "cocktail" of different types of medicines to maintain stability.

The FDA has approved of several drugs as mood stabilizers, including lithium, Lamictal, Depakote, anticonvulsants, and antipsychotic agents. Depakote is also used to prevent migraine headaches, and Lamictal is especially effective for treating persons on the "down" side of a manic-depressive cycle.

The wrong medication can cause problems that cannot be corrected. Be sure to ask about other medications, both over the counter and prescribed.

Unfortunately, all mood stabilizers have side effects. Lithium, for example, can cause shaking or tremors, acne and skin rashes, thirst and increased need to urinate, decreased function of the thyroid, kidney problems, and a cloudy thinking that can be most disturbing. Weight gain is also a common side effect of taking lithium. Patients on a lithium treatment course need to have blood tests several times a year to be sure that thyroid and kidney functions are normal.

Depakote also requires blood testing every three to six months to monitor for liver problems and toxicity. The FDA has put a black box warning on Depakote for pancreatitis and liver failure. Other side effects from Depakote include weight gain, sedation, hair loss, and polycystic (with multiple cysts) ovaries.

Bipolar patients are more likely than psychotic patients to suffer side effects.

As disconcerting as this list may seem, Depakote may have fewer negative effects than lithium.

The list of side effects for Lamictal begins with fatigue and includes dizziness, cognitive impairment (memory, logic lapses), and a rash known as Stevens-Johnson Syndrome that can be life threatening.

Here's a positive note: No blood tests are needed for patients taking Lamictal.

We have already discussed the side effects of antipsychotics. It is believed that bipolar patients are more likely to experience these side effects.

Mood Stabilizers (Anti-Manic & Anticonvulsants)

Relative Adverse-Effect Profiles

Agent	Usual Adult Dosage (mg/d)	Common Adverse Effects
Carbatrol, Equetro, Tegretol/Tegretol XR (carbamazepine)	800-1,200 epilepsy	dizziness, drowsiness, unsteadiness, nausea, vomiting
Eskalith (lithium carbonate) Lithobid Eskalith CR	1,800 acute 900-1,200 maintenance	nausea, fine hand tremor, polyuria, thirst, toxicity, diarrhea, vomiting, drowsiness, muscular weakness, lack of coordination
Deputing/ Depakote (valproic acid)	500-1,800	nausea, vomiting, diarrhea, abdominal cramps, sedation, tremor, weight gain, thrombocytopenia, increased liver function tests, hair loss
Symbyax (fluoxetine and olanzapine)	6-12 (olanzapine) 25-50 (fluoxetine)	edema, increased appetite, pharyngitis, somnolence, abnormal thinking, tremor, weight gain

Adapted from CNS News Special Edition December 2004

Stimulants

*I*n psychiatry, stimulants are used primarily to treat ADHD. The goal of treatment with stimulants is to improve individual performance academically and socially. Although children with ADHD may look hyperactive, their brains show a pattern of hypoactivity especially in the part of the brain called the anterior cingulate cortex. Medications that treat ADHD increase activity in this part of the brain.

Psychiatrists know they need to treat their patients early in their illness while their fragile self esteem may still be intact. For younger patients, obtaining a solid reputation at school requires early intervention so that basic skills are learned and social skills are allowed to develop.

Each person's daily patterns must be considered when setting a course of treatment. Monday may involve a trip to town and housework. Tuesday might be the day to pay bills and put in some time as a volunteer—and so on throughout the week. For students, a busy schedule of sports, studies, clubs, and social activities can turn a calendar into a complex pattern of social and academic challenges.

To assist in obtaining a complete and accurate profile, you can play a key role by talking to mom, dad, teacher, counselor, lunch room manager. For students the medication and dose may change by season, by sport, and in other ways.

All of us would like to improve our academic and social skills. From prescription drugs to illicit drugs sold on the street, stimulants are popular because they promise to deliver the boost in alertness and concentration that we crave. Probably the most famous prescribed stimulant is Ritalin. You are familiar with the street names of dozens of illicit stimulating drugs, such as "bennies," "uppers," "speed," "ice," "crack," "snow," and "meth."

Illicit use of stimulating drugs penetrates all classes of society, including professionals who revel in the higher levels of productivity and creativity that result. Taken carelessly, these drugs can become addictive, and many careers are ruined as a result of trying to support a costly and devastating drug habit.

Stimulants made their first appearance in the medical world in 1937 when the pioneer of psychostimulants, Charles Bradley, prescribed Benzedrine for children with severe behavior problems. Instead of running amok in the classroom, the children became interested in their schoolwork and wanted to learn more. They worked faster and more accurately and dubbed Benzedrine the "arithmetic pill" because of the dramatic improvement in their math performance.

Standing in awe of his own discovery, Bradley commented—

"To see a single dose of Benzedrine produce a greater improvement in school performance than the combined efforts of a capable staff working in a most favorable setting, would have been all but demoralizing to the teachers had not the improvement been so gratifying from a practical standpoint."

A half century went by after the introduction of Ritalin before children and others diagnosed with Attention Deficit Hyperactivity Disorder (ADHD) were treated with stimulants. Today controversy rages about the use of Ritalin and other stimulants for children and adults. Fortunately, fears of addiction and stunted growth by children being treated with stimulants are largely unfounded.

In the interest of public safety, The FDA has categorized Ritalin and amphetamines as Schedule II drugs that are as tightly regulated as are narcotics.

Schedule II drugs are closely monitored by the DEA.

Prescriptions for Schedule II drugs must be written on a special prescription pad that is difficult to copy or tamper with. All are monitored by the Drug Enforcement Agency (DEA), so the doctor can't just pick up the phone and authorize a prescription.

Cylert was a third type of stimulant available for many years. It was found to cause severe liver problems and was finally taken off the U.S. market in March 2005.

How stimulants work

You may be wondering how a stimulant can be helpful in treating a child with ADHD. We want the hyperactive child to calm down, not to become more excited. Do stimulants perk up a laid-back person and calm one who is in a frenzy?

Not at all. The mechanism works the same no matter what the condition may be. Stimulants work on increasing dopamine and norepinephrine. Researchers now think that increasing these neurotransmitters in the parts of the brain that allow people to pay attention to their impulses and control them is key to the successful treatment of ADHD.

People with ADHD are prone to a sense of worthlessness that can progress to depression. The goal in using stimulants in their treatment is to treat the person quickly before self esteem suffers and secondary problems occur.

Don't be too quick to conclude that a child should be treated for ADHD. Dad may think that Josh is a terror in danger of wrecking the house while Mom sees their son as a healthy bundle of energy. A teacher may be concerned about a child who seems to be giggling or talking all the time, while Grandma likes her little chatterbox just the way she is. Be sure that *social or academic functioning is impaired* and consider a variety of information sources dealing with the child's behavior problems before concluding that stimulants to treat ADHD are in order. In fact, the American Academy of Pediatrics requires the impairment to be observed in more than one domain (social, home, school, etc.) before treatment for ADHD is warranted.

Ritalin

Most stimulants prescribed today are in the Ritalin or the amphetamine families.

The chemical name for Ritalin is methylphenidate. Patented in 1950, Ritalin is the oldest and best known of all stimulants with methylphenidate as the active ingredient. Other drugs in the Ritalin family include sustained release and long-acting versions of Ritalin, Focalin (an isomer of Ritalin), Concerta, and Metadate. Members of the amphetamine family are Dexedrine, Adderall, Adderall XR (extended release), and Desoxyn.

A crucial fact about stimulants is their half life, the amount of time it takes for half the drug to leave the system. For Ritalin, the time period when the drug is effective is only three or four hours.

This poses a problem for a school-age child. To receive Ritalin's benefits throughout the school day and during after-school activities, a child would have to take a pill several times a day—not a good option for treating children with their busy school and play schedules. The whole issue of storing and accessing controlled drugs throughout the day can be a problem for the school. Additionally, any kid who pops pills throughout the day is likely to be the object of inquiries and ridicule.

A sustained release version of Ritalin (Ritalin SR) that lasts up to five hours has been released. A long-acting version (Ritalin LA) provides adequate coverage for eight hours, making it much easier for the child to take the medicine twice a day, once before leaving for school and, if needed, in the afternoon when school's out.

Sustained release Ritalin is easier for school-aged youngsters to take.

Studies show that the long-acting version of Ritalin delivers benefits that are similar to those of regular Ritalin but with fewer fluctuations and the convenience of fewer doses per day.

Another stimulant in the Ritalin family, Concerta, lasts eight to twelve hours, and Metadate works from five to eight hours.

Pharmaceutical companies are creative in coming up with novel delivery systems for their medicines. In the case of stimulants, coated tablets and time-release strategies result in medicines with actions that peak at different times and have different half lives.

Daytrana is the first patch approved by the government for the treatment of ADHD and is designed for children who can not (or will not) swallow pills. Daytrana is another methylphenidate (Ritalin) preparation that delivers the medication continuously over the nine-hour wear time with effects lasting as long as twelve hours.

The patch can be taken off earlier if a shorter duration is desired or if late-day side effects are bothersome.

Daytrana comes in 10, 15, 20, and 30 milligram strengths. It is recommended that patients start with the 10 milligram patch and titrate up, even if they were previously taking a methylphenidate drug.

Parents should be warned to dispose of the patch properly as it still contains quite a bit of drug. For example, the 30 milligram patch contains enough methylphenidate to release another 10 milligram over three hours.

Possible side effects include a mild skin irritation in addition to methylphenidate side effects already discussed.

Amphetamines

A leading amphetamine is Dexedrine, with a half life of three to four hours. Dexedrine Spansules contain timed-released "beads" that deliver benefits for up to eight hours. Half of the beads in a capsule are immediate release, delivering the medicine to the blood stream as soon as it is ingested. The other half are extended release beads covered with a sheath that delays release for four hours after the medicine is taken.

Another amphetamine stimulant is Adderall, available in regular formulation with a half life of three to four hours and an extended release (XR) version with up to nine hours of full effect.

Desoxyn is a methamphetamine stimulant that is used to treat obesity. It is the only stimulant approved by the FDA for treating people with a weight problem, although its use in weight loss is recommended only for those who have not been able to lose weight with other medications or programs. Only rarely is Desoxyn prescribed to treat ADHD.

Stimulants are approved by the FDA for treatment not only of ADHD but also of narcolepsy, a condition marked uncontrolled episodes of deep sleep. Stimulants are also prescribed off label for depression in individuals who have not been helped by other forms of treatment—and to help lessen fatigue and apathy associated with a variety of medical illness.

All stimulants have potential for abuse and unwanted side effects, not to mention public outcries against the "drugging" of our kids by people concerned about overprescribing these powerful medications.

Possible side effects associated with the use of stimulants

- Appetite suppression
- Insomnia
- Rebound irritability
- Headache
- Agitation
- Increased blood pressure
- Tics
- Liver problems (Cylert only)

Strattera (atomoxetine) is a non-stimulant medication that the FDA approved in 2002 for treating children and adults with ADHD. Strattera functions as a norepinephrine reuptake inhibitor, although it affects dopamine as well. Unlike stimulants, Strattera takes several weeks for its effect to become apparent. Problems often associated with stimulants such as unwanted weight loss due to appetite suppression and insomnia do not typically occur with Strattera. Of course, there is no free lunch. Strattera can cause sleepiness, nausea, and urinary retention.

There have been recent reports of Strattera-induced manic symptoms. This should not be too surprising, since its mechanism of action resembles that of some antidepressants. A number of medications not formally approved for treatment of ADHD are used successfully for many patients. These include Wellbutrin, an antidepressant (see page 69), tricyclic antidepressants, and clonidine, a medicine designed to control high blood pressure.

Acetyl-L-Carnitine, a nutrient used in the treatment of Alzheimer disease because of its positive effect on cognitive abilities, also shows promise in the treatment of ADHD. Manufactured by the body from amino acids, L-Carnitine shuttles long chain fatty acids into the mitochondria, the "furnace" of the cell. Within the furnace, fatty acids are broken down or burned and energy is produced. L-Carnitine is essential for the production of energy from fat. Trials suggest that the substance may be especially effective in treating children with uncontrolled impulses.

Sleep and Wakefulness

Around the clock, we're either asleep or awake, and it sometimes seems that people have as many problems staying awake as they do getting to sleep. More than seventy sleep disorders have been identified by health scientists, with insomnia as the most common sleep-related complaint. In terms of cost to society, however, staying awake on the job and on the road is an even greater concern.

With the discussion of sleep and wakefulness in this chapter, we merge into lifestyle issues that affect all of us. The ethical question immediately arises: Should we be taking drugs to deal with our poor choices in daily living?

The short answer is No. We should address our bad habits, trade them for good ones, and live as healthfully as we can without using medicine to reverse bad decisions. There will, however, always be a gap between what we "should" do and what ends up getting done.

> There will always be a gap between what we "should" do and what ends up getting done.

As an example, many of us fall short when it comes to good sleep habits because of illness, stress, and, in some cases, mental or physical disorders. Fatigue is the most common reason for disability in persons with depression. Addressing issues related to poor sleep is an important area of concern for persons involved in all of healthcare.

An estimated one out of thirty drivers is habitually sleepy, and sleepy drivers cause far more road mishaps than do inebriated drivers. One study reported that four out of ten motor vehicle crashes in New York were related to the fact that the driver fell asleep behind the wheel. We also know that people who work the graveyard shift are more likely to be involved in vehicle crashes.

Improving the quality of sleep can help prevent illnesses from worsening in people with a variety of health problems ranging from mental disorders to cancer. The benefits of sleep go beyond the sick bed. All of us need restful sleep. Adults need seven or eight hours a night, teenagers need about nine hours, and infants should sleep sixteen hours a day.

The sleep-wake cycle

The first step in dealing with sleep disorders is to understand the sleep-wake cycle. Early researchers found that even when isolated from all clues about what time of day it is, people tend to follow a sleep-wake cycle of approximately twenty-four hours. Apparently human beings are equipped with a built-in circadian rhythm mechanism for sleeping and waking.

Each half of the sleep-wake cycle depends on the other half to function properly. Being wide awake and energetic during the day helps you work and play hard so that you end the day ready to sleep. After a restful night sleeping, you wake up refreshed and energetic for another day.

Managing the sleep-wake cycle can be a challenge because physical illness, stress, pain, light, or noise can disrupt sleep and set you up for a day of sleepy exhaustion. This can become a vicious cycle leading to loss of productivity at work and other problems.

For many people, sleep problems go away on their own or with the help of simple practices such as cutting back on caffeine, going to bed at the same time every night, and avoiding alcohol.

For persons whose sleep problems cause significant distress, medication may be needed to help them get the sleep they need.

Hypnotics for sleep

Sedatives known as hypnotics work on either GABA or on histamine neurotransmitters. If you've ever taken an allergy pill you know that the "cure" for your sneezing and runny nose is an antihistamine. The problem is that in the brain histamines help keep you awake, so antihistamines inevitably make you sleepy. The reason the newer antihistamines such as Claritin are not likely to make you sleepy that they do not cross the blood-brain barrier to affect the histamines.

Barbiturates are sedative-hypnotic drugs that have been used to induce drowsiness since the 1860s. Barbituric acid, the base material of barbiturates, is a combination of urea and malonic acid and in itself does not affect the central nervous system. It was first synthesized on December 4, 1863, by Adolph von Bayer, the founder of the pharmaceutical firm by his name. He also synthesized aspirin, heroin, and many other compounds. The date of the discovery was the feast day of Saint Barbara, so von Bayer named his discovery "Barbara's urates" in her honor.

Barbiturates were named after the feast day of Saint Barbara.

The most common barbiturates are Nembutal (pentobartital) and Seconal (secobarbital). They are very rarely used in psychiatry but are still sometimes used to relax a patient before surgery or to control seizures. An overdose of barbiturates can lead to coma and death, and the combination of barbiturates and alcohol is particularly deadly. As if these problems aren't enough, barbiturates are highly addictive.

For these and other reasons, barbiturates are rarely prescribed today to help people with sleep disorders.

In response to these problems, pharmaceutical scientists developed a new category of sleep-aid drugs known as "benzos," short for benzodiazepines. (See page 84 for more about this class of medicines.) Examples of "benzo" sleep medicines are Halcion and Dalmane.

Halcion (triazolam) is a very short-acting benzo with a half life of only about one hour. Restoril (temazepam) remains effective for seven to eight hours, and Dalmane (flurazepam) is active in the system for up to thirty hours. Drug addicts often resort to benzos such as these when they want to "chill out" or come down from a drug-induced high.

Addicts use benzos to "chill out" after a high.

As effective as these drugs may be in bringing on sleep, they can be physically addictive and can cause uncomfortable symptoms when discontinued.

Because of this, new sleep aids have been developed. Non-benzos, as they are called, include Ambien (zolpidem), Sonata (zaleplon), and Lunesta (eszopiclone). A new version of Ambien—Ambien CR—was introduced in the U.S. in October of 2005. The manufacturer claims it gives people a hour or two more of sleep than Ambien does.

Ambien only takes a few minutes before its effects are felt and while it is not a narcotic, it is dangerous when used with alcohol. Sonata acts quickly and diminishes quickly as well, making it an ideal sleep aid for the person who wakes up at 3 a.m. and would like a few more hours of sleep before taking on the challenges of the day.

Lunesta is formulated to reduce insomnia by helping the person fall asleep more readily and stay asleep. Unlike other sleep aids mentioned in this section, Lunesta is approved to be used for up to six months.

Realize that at higher doses "non-benzo" medications come to act just like benzos.

Rozerem (ramelteon) is the first prescription sleep aid that works on melatonin receptors. The drug offers a new mechanism of action for insomnia, targeting two receptors in the brain, MT1 and MT2. These receptors are located in the brain's suprachiasmatic nuclei (SCN), known as the body's "master clock" because it regulates the 24-hour sleep-wake cycle. The MT1 receptor is thought to regulate sleepiness, while the MT2 receptor is thought to help the body shift easily between phases of day and night. Together, these receptors are believed to serve as key mediators of sleep in humans, encouraging the onset of sleep.

Antihistamines promote sleep.

Rozerem is a chronohypnotic because it works on the body's natural clock, compared with a sedative-hypnotic, which merely makes a person sleepy. A big advantage of Rozerem is that it cannot be abused. There is no risk of dependence or addiction.

Sleep aids at the local drugstore

What about over-the-counter sleep aids? The sleep-deprived customer can choose from dozens of products designed for another purpose but with the added benefit of helping the person sleep. For most of these products, antihistamines are the agents that bring about sleep as well as alleviating symptoms of allergies. Diphenhydramine is also marketed as Sominex and Unisom and is the sleep agent in Tylenol PM.

Controversy surrounds the use of the hormone melatonin as a sleep aid. Since is it classified as a dietary supplement and not as a drug, melatonin has not been rigorously tested or evaluated for effectiveness and possible side effects.

The FDA approves sleep aids for two reasons: (1) sleep onset, or falling asleep and (2) sleep maintenance, or staying asleep.

Common sleep aids

Sleep aid	Onset of action	Elimination half life	Adult dose
Sonata (zaleplon)	10-20 min	1.0 hrs	5-20 mg
Ambien (zolpidem)	10-20 min	1.5-2.4 hrs	5-20 mg
Ambien CR (zolpidem)	10-20 min	1.5-2.4 hrs	7.25-15 mg
Halcion (triazolam)	10-20 min	1.5-5 hrs	0.125 mg-0.25 mg
Restoril (temazepam)	45 min	8-20 hrs	7.5-30 mg
ProSom (estazolam)	15-30 min	20-30 hrs	0.5-2 mg
Dalmane (flurazepam)	15-30 min	36-120 hrs	15-30 mg
Xanax (alprazolam)	15-30 min	9-26 hrs	0.25-1 mg
Klonopin (clonazepam)	20-60 min	19-50 hrs	0.25-1 mg

Sleep aid	Onset of action	Elimination half life	Adult dose
Lunesta (eszopiclone)	15-30 min	6 hrs	1-3 mg
Rozerem	15-30 min	1-2.6 hrs	8 mg

Adapted from CNS News Special Edition December 2004

Coming soon

Soon you may see Hypnostat on the market, which is Halcion delivered as a spray through the nasal passages. Halcion is so fast-acting that the potential for abuse is real. Anticipating this, the manufacturer designed a computer chip to control the dose of the drug. Hypnostat should work even faster than a pill because it enters the brain directly from the nasal passages. The expected time interval from application to the onset of benefits is less than fifteen minutes.

The development of gaboxadol, a GABA-A agonist with the possible advantage of facilitating slow wave sleep, has been halted due to an unacceptable number of psychiatric side effects. This medicine dealt with the restorative part of sleep, promising to improve sleep quality as well as quantity. Aside from gaboxadol's side effects, the theory behind it is still quite controversial among sleep specialists. We will see what happens!

Sleep Aids (Antihistamines)

Pharmacokinetic Parameters

Agent	Usual Adult Dosage (mg/d)	Onset (min)	t½
Unisom SleepTabs (doxylamine)	25	30	N/A
Unisom Gel Tabs (diphenhydramine)	25-100	120-240	2-8

Adapted from CNS News Special Edition December 2004

Currently prescribed sleep agents and some investigational drugs work by targeting gamma aminobutyric acid (GABA) receptors, which are located throughout the brain. In pre-clinical studies, Rozerem has shown no affinity for GABA, opiate, or histamine receptors.

VEC-162 is a MT1 and MT2 receptor agonist under investigation by Vanda Pharmaceuticals for the treatment of insomnia and depression. In June 2006 positive results were reported showing a significant shift in circadian rhythm as measured by plasma melatonin levels.

Another new drug being used to treat insomnia is Eplivanserin (SR 46349), a $5\text{-HT}_{2A/2C}$ receptor antagonist. The 5-HT2 receptors are responsible for absorbing 5-HT (or serotonin) back into neurons. The antagonistic action of Eplivanserin allows serotonin to circulate longer in the body and in greater amounts. In March 2005, Sanofi-Aventis reported that Eplivanserin had successfully completed a trial for the treatment of chronic insomnia, and they are also interested in investing this compound for the treatment of fibromyalgia.

Wake aids

Getting enough sleep at night is not a guarantee for staying awake the next day. Only in recent years have we turned our attention to medicines that aid in alertness during the waking hours. Nearly all wake-promoting agents work on at least one of these three neurotransmitters: norepinephrine, dopamine or histamine.

Provigil (modafinil) is an interesting wake promoting agent that has been approved in the treatment of persons with symptoms of excessive sleepiness, including narcolepsy, sleep apnea, and problems of wakefulness due to night shift work, a condition with its own acronym, SWSD, for Shift Work Sleep Disorder. Only one pill a day may be needed to maintain an appropriate state of wakefulness without interfering with normal sleep at night.

The active metabolite of a drug called Olmifon (adrafinil), Provigil has been studied in Europe for over twenty years. Olmifon was originally approved in France for the treatment of elderly patients who were unable to concentrate or were experiencing symptoms of depression.

Provigil can help you stay awake and alert, but it is not a stimulant. Its exact mechanism is not fully understood, but Provigil is believed to increase histamine and orexin activation and possibly work through norepinephrine reuptake inhibition in the sleep promoting area of the brain. Interestingly, the mechanism of Provigil—whatever it may be—enhances arousal during wakefulness when norepinephrine and dopamine are already active but does not interfere with sleep when these neurotransmitters are quiet.[*]

Although its action seems to mimic that of amphetamine, it is not an amphetamine and because it is not a Schedule II medicine, a prescription can be phoned to the pharmacy. Side effects seem to be less common than with stimulants but may include headache, insomnia, and anxiety.

Off-label uses for Provigil include treatment of fatigue and sleepiness associated with depression and its treatment, multiple sclerosis, cancer and other conditions.

Currently in development is Nuvigil, an isomer of Provigil. Nuvigil seems to be somewhat longer lasting and shows promise for treatment of sleepiness and cognitive dysfunction.

---

* The reference for this fascinating research is a report by Clifford Saper and Thomas Scammell in Vol 27, No. 2004, pages 11-12 of *Sleep*.

Are Meds the Only Answer?

Should we look to prescription medications to solve all of our mental health problems? Is the subject of this book—psychotropic medications—the only route to relief from symptoms of mental disorders?

Emphatically not! Meds are only part of the solution.

Careful analysis based on the caregiver's knowledge and experience is vital in understanding the components of a person's distress. Patients deserve a high degree of expertise from their primary care provider. They don't need to see the person they are trusting for their care searching frantically for an opinion. "One of our son's doctors kept calling a colleague at a teaching university to see what he should do next," a parent commented about her son's experience. This kind of uncertain treatment should not be tolerated.

A good psychiatrist considers medications as one piece of the puzzle, and you will, too, as you evaluate the benefits and drawbacks of other options.

Nutrition. Diet seems like a good way to build a healthy brain, but no one has come up with a specific food or combination that does the trick. It is vital, however, for anyone with a mental disorder to eat as healthfully as possible to provide adequate nutrition for the brain and body. This means enjoying a varied diet with plenty of fruits and vegetables and maintaining a sensible weight. Neurotransmitters are made from amino acids, which come from dietary protein. The messengers of the brain require proper nutrition so that they can improve a person's mental health.

Exercise. All of us do better when we exercise regularly, and there is new evidence that the mind may benefit significantly from a lifestyle that includes vigorous physical activity. A study at Duke University found that sixty percent of persons suffering from depression became free of symptoms after exercising thirty minutes at a time three days a week for four months.

Psychotherapy. Psychotherapy, the "talking cure," continues to prove itself as an effective way to deal with psychological problems. Many types of psychotherapy and psychological counseling are available today to treat specific conditions. The therapist often prescribes medication in addition to one-on-one sessions, and studies show that the combination of talk therapy and medication is more effective in dealing with depression than either psychotherapy or medication alone.

Self-help groups. Self-help groups that focus on chemical and other addictions, depression, post-traumatic stress disorder, grief recovery, marriage problems and a wide range of other emotional problems can be especially helpful in dealing with mental disorders that are triggered or made worse because of lifestyle or social situations.

Alcoholics Anonymous adopted the globally accepted Twelve Step program in the 1930s to help members understand and control their addiction to alcohol. Today twelve step programs have been developed to deal with dozens of emotional and physical addictions as well as troublesome life situations. The structure and group support of these programs can be powerful tools to help individuals find their way through a morass of emotional problems.

Pets. For the person stricken with senility or extreme depression, something a simple as a puppy, a cat, or an aquarium of tropical fish can be comforting and therapeutic. Owning a pet has been shown to reduce symptoms caused by stress. One study found that petting a dog can lower blood pressure, and a study at City Hospital in New York found that heart patients with pets had a better recovery rate than those without. More than once, a patient of mine has shared fond thoughts of a cat, a dog, or even a goat that has helped bring meaning and purpose to his or her life.

Meditation and a sense of humor. Meditation, relaxation, and the cultivation of a humorous outlook on life are helpful ways of minimizing the consequences of stress and mental disorders.

This is just an introduction to the thousands of ways we can help people entrusted to our care develop a healthy mental outlook on life even when things look grim.

Patients learn from us, and we can readily administer the "medicine" of a smile and a cheerful attitude without a prescription. Of all the medications that can be prescribed, monitored, augmented, and evaluated, hope is undoubtedly the element worthy of the greatest acclaim. With modern developments in pharmacology it is possible to pave the road to mental health so that more people can experience improved mental performance and emotional stability. Nevertheless, it is hope that works the biggest miracles, not only for those we serve but also for ourselves as professionals in the healing arts.

"A leader is a dealer in hope."
—Napoleon Bonaparte

Listening to Those Who Know

*T*hrough the years I have learned a great deal about psychiatry from my medical classes, from seminars, from books and journals, and from rubbing shoulders with the best and brightest in my profession, but the most effective teachers of all have been my patients and their family members. People who are personally affected by mental illness in one form or another have an abundance of wisdom to share if we will take the time to listen.

"At fifteen I was just starting to come of age," a young man said. "I was depressed. I felt helpless. I was losing control of my life. It was a very hard time for me, and in my college years it only got worse. Then, because of a careful program of medication and therapy I was able to go from helplessness to control. I was one of the lucky ones."

"My parents have always been there for me," one of my outstanding successes told me. "I couldn't have come as far as I have without their support."

A father told me of a doctor who had put his daughter on Paxil, but her condition didn't change. "We called the doctor and told him it wasn't working, but the doctor didn't look at the research to see what the problem could be. Instead, he quickly ordered another medication, and within a week or two she became extremely hyper. She went from being mellow into total psychosis."

Another patient remembers what happened when he failed to receive any benefit from medicine prescribed for his psychosis. "A couple of days after taking the prescribed medication, I felt stressed, scared, unsafe," he said. "It wasn't working. My parents would call the doctor. 'He's still psychotic,' they said. So they upped the dosage. I began gaining weight. I was always tired and kept trying to lie down, but when I did I was nervous and agitated. Finally I was treated successfully at the Menninger Clinic. It felt so good when I realized I finally had my sanity back."

Try to understand the medicines you or a person you care for are taking and how they are supposed to help. "You don't have to be ugly about it," one of my patients said. "Just bring your doctor the literature you found on the web, or the printed material that comes when you fill the prescription and say, 'It says this...and I'm concerned about your decision.' "

"Be active in your treatment," one patient suggested. "If a new drug comes out to treat your condition, read all the info on the drug you can find. Look up the web site for the drug. Ask for literature with an explanation of the drug—what it does, what it doesn't do, what the side effects may be. Then talk to your doctor about it. Be an informed patient."

Be informed and active in your treatment.

I think all of my patients would agree that good communications with the doctor is an essential ingredient in mental healthcare. "If you're not communicating well with your doctor, you're not going to receive the right treatment," one of them said. "It's a matter of trust. You're the client, and your job is to give your therapist as much information as you can so that your doctor can work to protect you. You need as much information as possible."

The mother of a young person who struggled with mental illness for eight years told me how important it is to be open with the doctor. "Lots of times my husband or I would say, 'I don't want to bother her with that,' but we were always glad we could. If you don't have a doctor you can go to with all your concerns, you don't have a doctor. She never gave us the idea that it wasn't good to share a concern with her. I believe you have to feel like you can call the doctor when there's something you don't understand."

Patients know how important the doctor-patient relationship is in getting a handle on mental illness. One of my patients put it this way: "If that relationship is violated because your doctor's not giving you the information you need or isn't really listening to what you're saying, you might as well walk away because you aren't getting the care you need."

"Communicate with both sides," a patient I'll call Brandon said when I asked him what advice he'd like to give the caregiver who works with the medical doctor. "Try not always to be defending the person 'up there,' Brandon said. "Don't just say, 'the doctor says,' or 'that's what the doctor thinks.' Look out for the person's

> **Don't just say, "The doctor says..."**

health above all and be sure the advice they're getting is good advice. When you talk to that person 'up there' (the medical doctor), relay accurate information. Tell the doctor what you're observing. Don't hold anything back. As a patient you're with the caregiver a lot more than you're with the doctor. He needs your eyes and ears to know what's going on."

Parents are often the most important players in the success of a patient's course of treatment, and patients who have resumed a normal life never forget it.

"We don't choose mental illness to give our family a bad time," a patient I'll call Ashley said, "but that's what happens." Ashley was lucky that her parents stayed with her throughout the ordeal. Not every parent can handle the stress. "When I stopped and thought of all I'd put my parents through…I realized it was a damned lot, that they'd gone the extra mile and more for me."

The mother of a troubled teenager said, "It's hard to realize deep down that your child is suffering. The agony in your child's heart and mind is more than you can fathom. It doesn't do any good to blame yourself for the problem and even worse to blame the child. Try to remember that this youngster who is severely depressed, or thrashing about uncontrollably, or hyper one minute and dark the next—that this is the same person you loved all his or her life. You can help your child by showing that you care, and care deeply."

"That is so true," a patient said. "Step one is realizing that mental disorders are often the result of chemicals gone wild in the brain. It's not psychological, not something you choose. I guess you'd say that mental problems are a result of nature, not nurture."

Mental disorders result from chemicals in disarray.

The father of a patient who struggled with mental illness throughout adolescence and early adulthood suggests being careful about judging the ability of the psychiatrist to guide the treatment of the person.

"It's difficult for even a good psychiatrist to make a good diagnosis," he said. "I've heard that a typical case takes three stabs at a diagnosis before they get the 'right' one."

Patients know better than we do that medications are wonderful, but they're not everything. "Without the support of persons important in your life, it's almost impossible to get things straightened out," one of my patients told me.

School can make a huge difference for young people who are severely disturbed. "I had a great counselor in high school," a former patient recalled, "and I was lucky to have some great math teachers. But all in all, he commented, "being manic-depressive in school without diagnosis or treatment is like being openly gay in the military. The stigma of mental illness is huge. It was even worse then, but it's still there. Nobody likes a kid with mental problems."

For one of my former patients, the turning point came in high school when he began to see beyond his personal problems to his potential. "College was when school began to be fun for me," he said. "I loved college and had great teachers. Graduate school was tough at first, until I learned to focus on learning instead of grades and began really enjoying my classes. My grades took care of themselves."

Shame is still an almost visible component of going through emotional turmoil. "I remember a game we played in psychology class," a patient told me. "We had to pick which person got the kidney transplant and were assigned attributes for making the choice. One attribute was schizophrenia. I felt immensely ashamed because I'd faced that diagnosis and knew how horribly negative it was. 'Oh, my God,' I cried out from within, 'if I ever get a kidney transplant...'"

Shame accompanies emotional turmoil.

"A good psychiatrist has a good sense of humor," a patient commented, adding that it's hard sometimes to find anything amusing about mental illness, but a light-hearted optimism helps everybody.

Never underestimate the contribution mentally ill people can make to the family, the community, the country. "People with mental illness are dedicated people who are serving their country," a former patient observed.

Unfortunately, many people with mental disorders do not have the advantage of a highly skilled personal physician who can direct them to appropriate treatment. I recommend the National Alliance for the Mentally Ill as an organization that can benefit all victims of mental disease and their family members.

A challenge

"I've come to realize," one of my patients confided in me, "that I am a member of the mentally ill community who has stabilized, and I have a normal life now."

Whether you are a professional in the healing arts or simply a caring person, I challenge you to find a reward as great as that of seeing pure gratitude in the eyes of a person who has been released from mental anguish.

Encouraging Words

*I*n no other branch of medicine is the understanding and cooperation of the patient more important than in psychiatry. The patient's full cooperation is the most important single ingredient in the process of lessening the symptoms of emotional and psychiatric distress. The insights of the patient help determine the diagnosis, and the patient's response to treatment determines the direction of the course.

Every time I see a patient of mine reach an improved state of behavior or achieve a higher degree of peace of mind, I know that much of the credit for this success belongs to the patient.

In this chapter I share tips and suggestions especially for people who turn to mental health professionals for advice and wisdom in coping with mental disorders. Our goal is for each individual to have a rewarding experience with the psychiatrist, other mental healthcare providers, and counselors.

Building trust

Never forget that a good doctor-patient relationship is founded on trust. Some tips that can help build a trusting relationship:

1. **Check credentials.** Don't hesitate to ask about the provider's academic and medical credentials, background and experience treating people with problems similar to yours.

2. **Trust your instincts.** During that first office visit you will instinctively know whether or not the person you

are seeing is someone you can respect and someone who will listen to you. If you feel extremely nervous or unsure about the doctor, look for someone else who can help you.

Be a partner

The journey to mental health is an exploration of discovery. Think of yourself as a partner with the doctor on this journey. Some specific suggestions:

1. **Don't hold back information.** Tell your doctor what's working. Your role is helping your doctor focus on what has gone wrong and what is working for you. You can help your doctor make good decisions based on your honest and full disclosure.

2. **Know what's going on.** Read books or search on the Internet to find out more about your situation and learn about the drugs your doctor may be prescribing for you. Being a well-informed patient will help you discuss your treatment plan with your doctor.

3. **Be wary.** Not all information in print or on the Web is accurate, and some is harmful. Your doctor can help you evaluate news reports, testimonials, and other documents related to your situation. You might even be able to share a tip or a suggestion that will be helpful to your care provider.

Be business like

Learn how to combine a warm and friendly attitude with a business-like atmosphere. Think of your relationship as an unwritten contract guiding both you and your doctor in get-

ting the most out of the experience. Some specific suggestions that may be helpful:

1. **Be on time.** Always be on time for your appointments.
   Respecting your doctor's schedule and being ready to
   begin your visit at the agreed time will put you on the
   right track.

2. **Answer the questions.** Provide all information
   requested honestly and completely. You will probably
   be given a rather lengthy form and asked to check
   descriptions that apply to you. Don't hold anything
   back.

3. **Give information in writing.** Instead of telling the
   doctor what medications you're taking or bringing the
   containers with you, make an address-sized label for
   each prescription or over-the-counter drug you're
   taking. Write down the name of the drug, the dose, and
   how often it is taken. The doctor can place these labels
   in your file and won't need to take the time to write
   down the details.

Example of label for the patient to give to the doctor

Effexor XR 300 mg in am	Synthroid 75 mcg in am
Lipitor 20 mg	Claritin as needed
Calcium 500 mg 2/d	Centrum 1 daily

4. **Ask questions.** In a business-like way ask questions
   such as, "How do we know this?" "How will this
   medicine affect my sleep (sex life, weight, etc.)?" or
   "How long do you think it will be before I start feeling
   better?"

5. **Follow the prescription.** Take medications as prescribed. Some of the medicines that affect the way your brain sends messages take days or even weeks before they take effect. You need to have a "therapeutic" level of the medicine in your blood stream for them to be effective. Your pharmacist will give you printed information when you pick up your prescription. Read these product sheets carefully and call the doctor's office if you don't understand something.

6. **Ask for test results.** Blood tests, urine tests, and even an MRI or strictly psychological tests may be ordered. You have every right to know how you did on the tests, what they show, what the normal ranges are and how the test results affect your treatment.

7. **Report side effects.** Tell your doctor about any side effects. If you start taking medicine and begin to feel pain in your stomach, rapid heart beat, or other strange sensations, assume it was your medicine and call the office right away. Side effects are not rare, and there are usually other drugs that will be just as effective without causing problems.

8. **Come prepared.** Make a list of questions before you arrive at your appointment. Write down the bad feelings or symptoms you've been experiencing.

9. **Record your visit.** Ask if it's okay with your physician and if it is, take notes during your visit or turn on a tape recorder. If this is hard for you to do, ask your doctor if it's okay for a family member or friend to come with you to the appointment or who can talk to you afterwards about your recommendations.

10. Use e-mail. A growing number of physicians, including many psychiatrists, encourage their patients to let them know how they're doing by sending e-mail. Be sure to ask first before using this method of communication with your provider.

All patients and recipients of prescription medication should have an active interest in their care and treatment. Don't hesitate to ask questions and be informed.

Understand Your Rights

Patients in America have rights that are spelled out and guaranteed by law. Here are some of your rights as a patient.

1. **The right to choose another doctor.** You don't have to go to court or pay a severance fee to dismiss your doctor. If you aren't satisfied with the care you are receiving, don't trust your doctor, or just don't like him or her, you don't have to remain a patient. Find another care giver.

2. **The right to be your doctor's partner.** We've already talked about the importance of having a solid business relationship with your doctor. This relationship gives you the right to ask any questions about your care that are important to you. There are no "stupid" questions.

3. **The right to know what else is available.** There is almost always more than one way to treat your symptoms. You have the right to know about other ways, even if they are not covered by insurance or are not considered "traditional" medicine.

4. **The right to refuse treatment.** If your doctor suggests a treatment you don't want such as electrical shock therapy for severe depression, politely say that you choose not to have this procedure. You may have to sign a form to relieve the doctor of any legal liability, but you don't have to undergo any treatment you choose not to endure.

5. **The right to leave a healthcare facility.** Even if your doctor says you need to be hospitalized or cared for in a controlled setting, you do not have to follow these orders. The only exception is that your legal guardian may make a decision to admit you to a hospital or other care facility if your age or mental state does not allow you under the laws of your state to make your own decisions.

6. **The right to your medical records.** You have the right to have photocopies of all of your medical records, although there may be a copying charge for making copies of the pages.

Patient to patient

I asked some of my patients if they had advice they'd like to share with other persons suffering from mental disorders. You might be able to pass some of these perspectives on to people you know are struggling with mental health issues.

The big picture. "You have to look at the big picture, and it is often hard to deal with facts appropriately," one of them said. "Nevertheless, you need to learn everything you can. If a doctor is being careless with meds, he is not a good doctor. Look at the literature for the prescribed medication. Learn the recommended dose and how fast it kicks in. Consult with other doctors. And don't be afraid to speak up when you see discrepancies."

Psychiatrists do make mistakes. Our patients occasionally remind us that even psychiatrists with perfect credentials make mistakes. "Once while I was being treated away from home I was stressing out," a patient recalled, "but not that much. My parents and I wanted to change medication because I was having trouble concentrating. So the doctor took me from Topamax to Depakote to see if that would help. The problem was that the doctor upped the meds too fast. The dose was 1,000 milligrams, and my parents insisted on his calling my psychiatrist at home. 'That's a crisis dose,' my psychiatrist told him. 'Don't give that dose.' "

Find the right psychiatrist for you. "If you are not getting the care you need, try to find another doctor," a patient of mine told me when I asked her what she thought her options were when she wasn't making progress. "It's not easy, but you have to have a psychiatrist who is on top of things. Yes, it's important to be seeing a psychiatrist, a person with special education and training in treating mental illness, but that's not enough. It has to be a good psychiatrist."

What is a good psychiatrist?

The Accreditation Council for Graduate Medical Education has identified six core competencies for physicians. A good psychiatrist is one whose expertise is of a high quality in patient care, medical knowledge, practice-based learning and improvement, interpersonal and communication skills, professionalism, and a systems-based practice that looks at the whole person and not just the specific problem that brings the patient to the care provider.

In more mundane terms, a good psychiatrist is coach and co-pilot, guide and mentor, teacher and example.

Resources for self-education

Local chapters of national organizations are dedicated to the promotion of mental health and Internet addresses are available where appropriate information can be obtained.

Share this book with those you feel would benefit from its facts and explanations.

Other possibilities—

NAMI. The National Alliance for the Mentally Ill (www.nami.org) is the "nation's voice on mental illness" and provides a wealth of services and information about mental illness, including a national convention every June.

Group support. Look for support groups in your community for persons affected by mental illness. If you don't find any, start one. Social ties in coping with these problems are especially valuable.

Diet and exercise. Patients who follow a healthy diet and exercise regularly will do better with any treatment program. Develop a routine that places physical health and well being at a high priority.

Be a partner. Most of all, see yourself as a partner in the mental health team along with family members and others directly affected by the mental illness.

When it comes to mental healthcare, the patient is always in the driver's seat. Learn to work with family members, physicians, counselors and others as you become more and more capable of taking charge of your own destiny.

Glossary

ADHD or ADD. Attention Deficit Hyperactivity Disorder. A common problem marked by poor concentration, restlessness, and inability to complete tasks. Adults as well as children are affected by this disorder.

AMPA. One of three glutamate receptors. The others are NMDA and Kainate.

bioequivalence. A characteristic of a drug that has the same chemical composition and accessibility to the body as another drug. Generic drugs are required by the FDA to be bioequivalent to the original medication.

anxiolytics. Antianxiety pharmaceutical agents that work primarily on serotonin and GABA neurotransmitters.

bipolar disorder. A problem involving persistent and disruptive mood swings known as "manic" or "depressive."

ECT. Electroshock therapy. A patient undergoing ECT experiences a seizure caused by electric shock delivered to the brain. ECT is rarely used but is often effective in cases of severe depression.

EPS Extrapyramidal syndrome. A condition that can range from a general state of restlessness to muscular spasms of the neck, eyes, tongue, or jaw.

FDA. Food and Drug Administration. Federal body that works to assure the safety and effectiveness of drugs, medical devices, and other products. All prescription drugs must be approved by the FDA before they can be marketed in the U.S.

GABA.   Gamma Amino Butyric Acid. An inhibitory transmitter that tends to calm and sooth, acting in an opposing way to glutamate.

GAD.   Generalized Anxiety Disorder. Chronic free-floating anxiety lasting more than six months.

histamine.   A neurotransmitter that lessens the effect of allergies and inflammation. In the brain, histamine influences sleep and wakefulness, hormones, cardiovascular control, food intake, and memory formation.

isomer.   A chemical with the same formula as another chemical but with a different arrangement of molecules and atoms within the chemical and a resulting effect that is different. Darvon and Novrad are examples of isomers. Darvon relieves pain while Novrad is used to control coughing.

MAO and MAOI.   Mono-amine oxidase (MAO), is an enzyme capable of rendering serotonin, dopamine, and norepinephrine dysfunctional. Drugs that interfere with these attacks are known as MAO Inhibitors or MAOI.

OCD.   Obsessive-compulsive disorder. A condition in which the brain seizes on a certain thought or urge and won't let go. Hand washing, repeating phrases, or sensing impending doom are examples of OCD behaviors.

psychotropic medications.   Medications that can bring healing by influencing the way the mind works.

reuptake.   The process of returning a substance to the cell that originated it.

SAD.   Seasonal Affective Disorder. A sense of depression or sadness that occurs during winter months when sunlight is less plentiful.

SCN. Suprachiasmatic nuclei. Home in the brain for MT1 and MT2 receptors and the location of the body's "master clock" that regulates the 24-hour sleep-wake cycle.

SNRIs. Serotonin norepinephrine reuptake inhibitors. The "N" represents norepinephrine.

SSRIs. Selective Serotonin Reuptake Inhibitors. Drugs that make serotonin more available by blocking the return (reuptake) of serotonin back to its presynaptic cells.

stereochemistry. See isomer. Stereochemistry is the mirror image arrangement of atoms in two chemically identical substances.

Stevens-Johnson Syndrome. A potentially fatal skin disease that rarely results as a reaction to some drugs, including Lamictal, a mood stabilizer.

SWSD. Shift Work Sleep Disorder. A state of constant disruption of sleep that results in excessive sleepiness or inability to sleep. People who work night shifts are especially vulnerable.

synapse. The transition point between two neurons. Vesicles in the synapse are packed with neurotransmitters waiting to be deployed.

tardive dyskinesia. A possible side effect of conventional antipsychotics. A person with this condition twitches or engages in other meaningless motions.

Learn More

This short book gives only a bare introduction to the exciting and rapidly changing field of psychotropic medications. I hope I've helped whet your appetite and that you are eager to learn more. Here are my suggestions for expanding your understanding of medications used in psychiatry.

I recommend all books and articles by Stephen Stahl, M.D., especially *Essential Psychopharmacology: The Prescriber's Guide*, 2nd edition, Cambridge University Press.

A scholarly but readable book with a comprehensive bibliography is *Psychopharmacology and Psychotherapy: A Collaborative Approach,* Michelle B. Riba, M.D., and Richard Balon, M.D. American Psychiatric Press.

You definitely should read *Prozac and the New Antidepressants: What You Need to Know about Prozac, Zoloft, Paxil, Luvox, Wellbutrin, Effexor, Serzone, Vestra, Celexa, St. John's Wort, and Others.* This is a candid and interesting treatment of antidepressant medications that are new on the horizon. By William S. Appleton, M.D., Penguin Group.

The Complete Guide to Psychiatric Drugs: Straight Talk for Best Results, by Edward Drummon, M.D., provides an encyclopedic view of the hundreds of drugs we now prescribe. John Wiley & Sons, Inc.

Other good sources: *Clinical Psychopharmacology Made Ridiculously Simple* by John Preston and James Johnson, MedMaster, Inc. *Neuroscience for the Mental Health Clinician,* Steven R. Pliszka, Guilford Press. *The Mind Within the Net,* Manfred Spitzer, MIT Press.

About the Author

Leslie Pedersen Lundt, M.D., received her undergraduate degree from Johns Hopkins University and her medical degree from Rush Medical College. She trained in psychiatry at the California Pacific Medical Center in San Francisco where she was Chief Resident and had additional training in addiction medicine at the Haight Ashbury Clinic. Dr. Lundt is board certified in psychiatry, addiction medicine and addiction psychiatry.

Dr. Lundt has practiced psychiatry and addiction medicine for two decades. She has a private clinical practice in Boise, Idaho, where she treats children, adolescents and adults. In addition, she has conducted numerous clinical research trials as a primary investigator. Dr. Lundt serves as a consultant to the media and various pharmaceutical companies. She is an affiliate faculty member of Idaho State University.

Education is a vital part of Dr. Lundt's professional and personal life. She directs Foothills Foundation, a non-profit educational group dedicated to teaching the public and other medical professionals about mental health topics. In addition, she co-founded a school for gifted children where she serves as admissions and curriculum director. Dr. Lundt lectures extensively and is well-known for her engaging and informative presentations. Special interests of Dr. Lundt include women's mental and reproductive health, psychopharmacology and addiction psychiatry.

Index